A Guide to Practical Procedures in Medicine and Surgery

H. A. F. Dudley, CBE, ChM, FRCS (Ed.), FRACS, FRCS
Professor of Surgery

J. R. T. Eckersley, FRCS
Orthopaedic Registrar

S. Paterson-Brown, FRCS (Ed.), FRCS
Surgical Registrar

Illustrations by Gillian Lee, FMAA, AIMBI
Medical and Biological Illustrator

Heinemann Medical Books

Heinemann Medical Books
An imprint of Heinemann Professional Publishing Ltd
Halley Court, Jordan Hill, Oxford OX2 8EJ

OXFORD   LONDON   SINGAPORE
NAIROBI   IBADAN   KINGSTON

First published 1989

British Library Cataloguing in Publication Data
Dudley, Hugh, *1925–*
   A guide to practical procedures in
   medicine and surgery.
   1. Medicine. Surgery. Techniques
   I. Title.   II. Eckersley, J.R.T.
   (J. Rupert. T.)   III. Paterson-Brown,
   S. (Simon) 617'.9

ISBN 0 433 00058 9

Typeset by Scarborough Typesetting Services
Printed in Great Britain by
LR Printing Ltd, Crawley, Sussex

Contents

Preface

For many years, the senior author of this book has been trying formally, both by a publication now out of print[1] and in our little manual for house staff[2], as well as informally by exhortation, to give instruction about the way so-called 'minor' procedures should be carried out. He has said time and again 'don't do it any old way; do it *my* way.' Sometimes, his staff have listened to him, and oral tradition has carried his ideas through many generations of junior staff in the Academic Surgical Units of Monash University at Alfred Hospital in Melbourne and St Mary's Hospital, London. However, he and his junior colleagues have come to feel that it is time to bring together these procedures in a pocket book, which like *A Guide for House Surgeons and Interns in the Surgical Unit*, could instruct students and recently qualified doctors in what we believe is best practice.

The text, we hope, includes all that junior staff should be asked to do. However, it goes a little beyond this into what they may have to *understand* even if the procedure has been performed by someone else. In this regard, we may not have gone far enough and we would welcome any suggestions for future editions.

Manual skills amongst junior staff are sometimes rudimentary and, when present, are often discounted. We believe that with adequate instruction, which we hope this book provides, and sympathetic training from the more experienced, students (under supervision) and house officers can safely perform quite invasive procedures of critical value in patient management. The geographically isolated general practitioner may also find this volume useful on occasion. We think it is best acquired during the student years and should be read and used in conjunction with *A Guide for House Surgeons and Interns in the Surgical Unit*.

We have had the special privilege of working closely with the artist Mrs Gillian Lee whose involvement in our book has made her an associate author. The outcome owes a great deal to her ability to make sense of our scrawls and to organize the graphics into a coherent whole.

Hugh Dudley, Simon Paterson-Brown, and Rupert Eckersley
Academic Surgical Unit, St Mary's Hospital, London W2 1NY

1. Dudley H. A. F. (1958). *Principles of General Surgical Management.* Edinburgh: Churchill Livingstone.
2. Fraenkel G., Dudley H., Ludbrook J., eds. (1987). *A Guide for House Surgeons and Interns in the Surgical Unit*, 8th edn. London: Heinemann Medical Books.

Acknowledgements

We gratefully acknowledge the help and advice given to us not only by our own colleagues in the Academic Surgical Unit but also those from other departments within St Mary's Hospital:

Anaesthetics	Dr Gary Symons
	Dr Jenny Jones
	Dr Henrietta Hill
	Dr Martin Read
	Dr Mike Ewart
Gastro-enterology	Dr Ian Barrison
Urology	Mr John Heatherington
Cardiology	Dr Phil Thomas
	Dr Mark Dixon
Histopathology	Dr Terry Cook
Accident and Emergency	Mr Robin Touquet
	Sister Proudfoot and the nursing staff

We would also like to thank Butterworths for giving us permission to reproduce some of the figures in Chapter 2, and the British Medical Journal for giving us permission to reproduce the figures on resuscitation in Chapter 5.

General principles

Sterility and practical procedures

Since Lister's introduction of the antiseptic concept in the 1860s and its refinement into *asepsis* thereafter, the doctor has always looked upon his role as protecting the patient from the risks of introducing infective agents during a procedure which breaches body defences. However, a new dimension has been added with the increasing recognition that body secretions in general, but blood in particular, can be inoculated into the operator and so transmit diseases such as hepatitis and acquired immunodeficiency syndrome (AIDS). We will discuss the precautions in relation both to the patient and to the medical team.

MANAGEMENT OF THE PATIENT

Ideally every procedure, however minor, should be carried out in an environment which is of the highest level of cleanliness with the best possible standard of aseptic surgical technique. However, this counsel of perfection is neither pragmatically justified by the risks nor is it logistically possible. We distinguish three levels:

(1) Very minor procedures – e.g. venepuncture, setting up a peripheral infusion, fine needle aspiration and needle biopsy of superficial lesions.
   Environment required: a clean room or ward
   Isolation of the area: minimal, so that sterile objects cannot be laid down at will
   Surgical preparation: clean but not sterile hands; no gloves – but see below for special circumstances
   Surgical technique: 'no touch' – i.e. the hands do not come into contact with any sterile material or surface.
(2) Minor ward or treatment room procedures which carry an increased risk if sepsis occurs – e.g. lumbar puncture, percutaneous great vein puncture, peripheral venous cut-down.
   Environment required: a treatment room or operating room with good quality lighting
   Isolation of the area: complete draping
   Surgical preparation: full scrub (see below); gloves, gown and mask
   Surgical technique: 'no touch' as far as possible.
(3) All other procedures should be carried out in the operating suite where there are full sterile precautions, good lighting and, most important, *back-up* if things go wrong.

Skin preparation

It is now generally recognized that the skin cannot be sterilized because of resident organisms in sweat glands and hair follicles or those lying under protective epidermal scales. However, this is not a reason for laxity. Skin areas involved in minor procedures should be physically clean and shaved immediately before the procedure (not some hours before as this may result in abraded areas which become colonized with bacteria). A sufficient area should be cleared so that adhesive tape used at the end of the procedure is not placed on hair. A single application of an antiseptic is then made. The following are suitable:

Chlorhexidine gluconate(1.5%)/*cetrimide*(0.5%) aqueous solution – usually known as Savlon (ICI)
Povidone iodine(10%) in alcohol – Betadine (Napp)
Chlorhexidine gluconate(0.5%) in 70% alcohol – often known as Hibitane (ICI)
Iodine(2.5%) in 90% alcohol

Isopropyl alcohol is also commonly available as wipes but is a de-fatter rather than an antiseptic.

PREPARATION FOR THE OPERATOR

You are strongly advised to seek active immunization against hepatitis B because your risk as a doctor of acquiring this potentially fatal disease although low is real. There is currently no immunization available against AIDS. You are justified in taking additional precautions to protect yourself from blood or other secretions in patients who:

(1) have AIDS
(2) are known to have antibodies against HIV
(3) are thought to be in a rather ill-defined 'high risk' group – male homosexuals and intravenous drug abusers.

These additional precautions are gloves to protect your hands during *any* contact with the patient and some form of eye protection against splash – glasses or goggles. Try not to let these additional precautions alarm the patient.

Clean hands

A study at a distinguished teaching hospital in the USA showed that only 20% of staff washed their hands after any form of contact with patients in an intensive care unit. Make it a firm rule of your own practice to wash after any contact, either social or professional, with any patient.
Before a minor procedure, scrub your nails briefly and wash for one minute with soap and water. Dry your hands meticulously on paper towel.
For a full hand preparation:

(1) Check that your nails are physically clean
(2) Wash them under running water for thirty seconds
(3) Scrub the nails for one minute with a firm brush
(4) Wash your hands and forearms for one and a half minutes
(5) Dry hands and forearms with a sterile towel and put on a gown and gloves.

Masks

There is a difference of opinion about the need to wear masks for *any* surgical procedure but it is conventional still do do so. There is no doubt about the oronasal carriage of pathogens by some, though not all, people.

3

What is more in question is whether – short of sneezing, coughing or spitting into the operative field – these organisms gain access to or cause infection in a surgical wound. The best course of action is to look upon masks as a sign of surgical ritual, an overall indication of the need to maintain high standards. Needless to say that, if they are to be any good at all, they must be worn to cover the nose but not the eyes.

GENERAL ADVICE ON MINOR PROCEDURES

Small procedures which the operator regards as minor can still be very trying for the patient. Make sure that he or she is as comfortable as possible and say what you are doing or going to do next. Minimize draping around the head to avoid a feeling of claustrophobia and, if you are capable of it, keep up a flow of distracting conversation. Get yourself in a relaxed position; sit down whenever you can. Make sure the light is good. Check that you have everything you think you will need before you begin. At all times, take especial care of sharps – needles, knives and scissors – to avoid accidental injury to yourself or your patient.

DRESSINGS

Punctures, except those made with a very fine needle, should be covered with a small, adhesive and preferably waterproof dressing. Do not forget to tell the patient to remove this at 48 hours, otherwise you may see him or her again a week later with a rather dirty and mangled piece of material hanging on grimly by its remaining adhesive.

Incisions, except those on the face which are better left exposed, are dressed with a dry gauze cover which is not waterproof so that the wound underneath can dry out. Exceptions may need to be made to this rule with wounds in areas that will inevitably be wetted.

There are only rarely indications for 'non-adherent' dressings, which are more expensive than plain gauze. Occasionally, a raw granulating area needs to be dressed repeatedly but, in that it wets the dressing itself, non-adherence is built in. Donor sites for skin grafts are conventionally covered with 'tulle gras' (paraffin jelly impregnated gauze), but this only encourages nurses and others to look at the area before it is healed. It is far better to use dry gauze and leave the area strictly alone until the dressing comes off of its own accord at about 10 days. Some plastic surgeons use plastic film (Opsite, Smith and Nephew), but this is quite difficult to manage unless you are expert.

Plastic adherent film is also useful for areas that it is desirable to keep under observation – e.g. the insertion point of a central venous catheter (p. 49).

All tissue removed from a patient should be submitted for histological examination whatever the apparent nature of the lesion. Temptation to save the pathologist extra work by discarding even the most benign looking naevus or cyst must be avoided.

FIXATIVE

Specimens usually need to be placed in fixative after removal, the nature of which will depend on the histological examination required. A 10% solution of formalin in saline is used for standard sections but some tissues and tests require a different fixative or may be best submitted fresh or frozen. It is therefore important to have close liaison with the local histology department as to the most appropriate method of handling different specimens. If the standard formalin in saline solution (formal saline) is used, then there should be 10 times as much fluid as specimen by volume. Less fixative than this will result in a prolonged or incomplete fixation of the specimen and will delay examination.

PREPARATION

Small mucosal samples, such as a rectal biopsy, should be removed from the biopsy forceps with the point of a 21G needle and placed onto a piece of blotting paper before immersion in fixative. This helps to prevent excessive distortion of the biopsy, which can make subsequent examination difficult.

Specimens for which information concerning clearance margins is required must be adequately oriented and labelled. This may necessitate pinning the specimen onto a cork board or attaching a suture to part of it before placing it in the fixative.

LABELLING

It is the responsibility of the surgeon to ensure that both the container and the accompanying form are adequately labelled. A concise clinical history and any specific request should always be included to help the pathologist in his quest for a diagnosis.

Chapter 2

Basic surgical technique

Basic surgical technique

There are many books which will tell you how to undertake the steps of an operation or procedure. It is less easy to find instructions on the 'basics' or how to handle surgical tools – what North American surgeons call *tissue technique* – and you are usually left to acquire this by observation and imitation; the outcome may be that you succeed only in picking up other people's bad habits.

Always try to study your own performance in order to eliminate unnecessary manoeuvres. Try to avoid all repetition. Get things right the first time – do not pick up a skin flap and then put it down again while you put the needle holder in the right place. It sounds trivial perhaps but it happens all the time.

INSTRUMENTS

You will use only a few basic instruments for the simple things you do as a junior or senior house officer: a knife, dissecting forceps, scissors, other ring-handled instruments such as artery forceps (known by a wide variety of names, e.g. points, snaps, haemostats, clips) and needle holders.

Knife

There are two grips: external (Fig. 2.1) and internal (Fig. 2.2). For minor surgery, the internal grip – which is similar to that used in handling a pen – is delicate and easily controlled. However, start an incision by using the external grip to puncture the skin with the point of the knife through the tough dermis. Remember that you can use a knife to cut tissues only if they are held on the stretch – use the other hand or tissue forceps to achieve this.

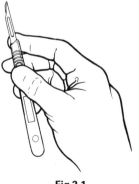

Fig 2.1

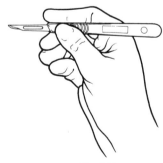

Fig. 2.2

Dissecting forceps

There are two kinds: toothed (Fig. 2.3A) for gripping tissues such as skin and fascia, which contain a large amount of collagen and are thus resistant to tear; and plain (Fig. 2.3B) for delicate tissues such as bowel. Dissecting forceps are nearly always held in the left hand with an internal *triangular* grip (Fig. 2.4) and can be nestled in the palm of the hand when not in use (Fig. 2.5).

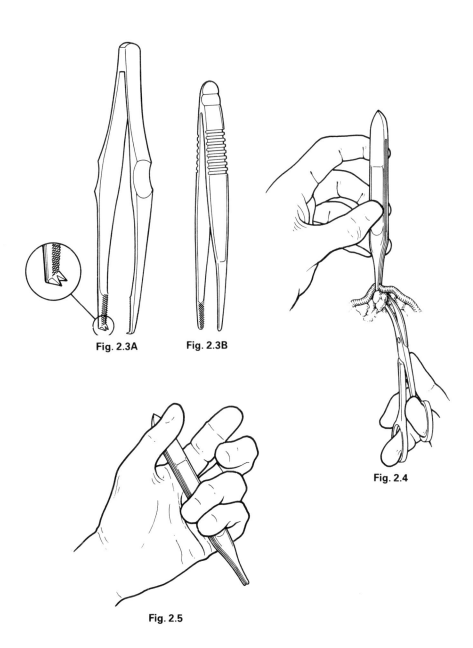

Fig. 2.3A   Fig. 2.3B

Fig. 2.4

Fig. 2.5

Ring-handled instruments

All of these should be used with the hand in partial or complete supination (Fig. 2.6A); if the hand is turned into pronation (Fig. 2.6B), it is more difficult to see the area which is being worked on and also there is less flexibility in controlling the position of the point of the instrument. Always use the thumb and *fourth* finger to hold the two rings because this gives better control. Scissors work because of the apposition of the blades at the point where they cross. To ensure that this is at a maximum, press upward on the right hand limb with the thumb and pull down with the fourth finger (Fig. 2.7); a left hander has to do the opposite unless the scissors are specially made (rare). All ringed instruments can be lodged in the palm (Fig. 2.8). For a method of modifying the grip on a ringed needle holder see p. 17.

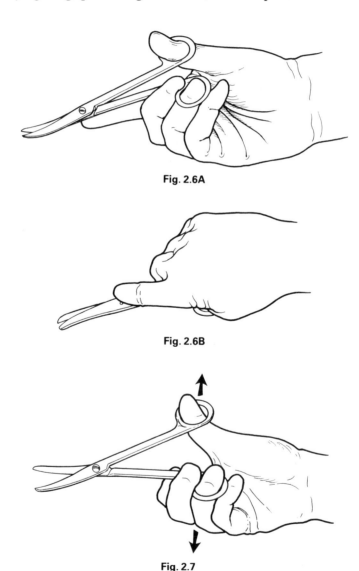

Fig. 2.6A

Fig. 2.6B

Fig. 2.7

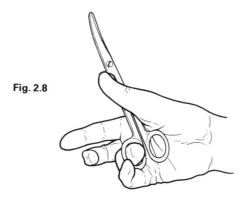

Fig. 2.8

Removing ratchet ring-handled instruments

This is often necessary when assisting at operations. Use either of the techniques shown (Figs. 2.9A and B). Do not put the fingers deeply into the rings. Practise until you are proficient with either hand.

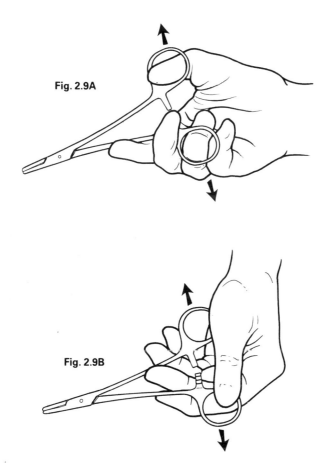

Fig. 2.9A

Fig. 2.9B

11

Knot tying

Ask an experienced surgeon to show you how to tie both one-handed and two-handed knots – this is far better than trying to learn from diagrams. The best surgeons can tie knots by both techniques with either hand as the *active* one, and that standard should be your aim. The steps of tying with a needle holder are shown in Fig. 2.10A–E.

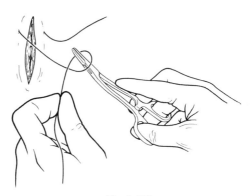

Fig. 2.10A

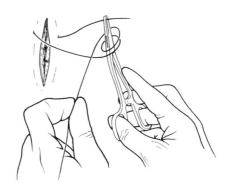

Fig. 2.10B

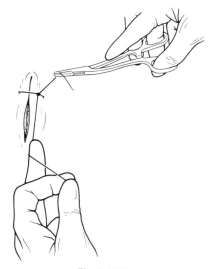

Fig. 2.10C

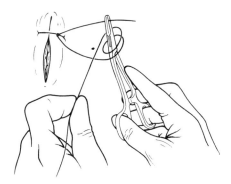

Fig. 2.10D

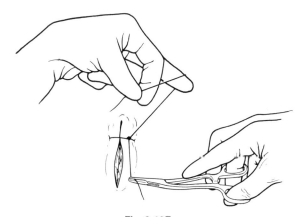

Fig. 2.10E

Simple wound excision and closure

Most civilian wounds in accident and emergency or after admission in patients with minor trauma are easy to deal with. Surgical pride, however, should make you wish to produce the best possible result. Before treatment is undertaken, you must of course be absolutely sure of the physical examination with particular reference to blood and nerve supply beyond the injury.

(1) Shave the immediate surrounding area using a disposable scalpel blade or razor (Fig. 2.11). Not only does this delineate the injury better but also it makes it easier for you to achieve precise apposition.

(2) Clean and isolate the area (see p. 2). General dirt should be removed from the surrounding skin with a soft nail brush and copious plain soap and water.

(3) Infiltrate local anaesthetic (see p. 23).

(4) Gently explore the wound using a blunt instrument such as the tip of curved dissecting scissors or a non-toothed forceps. Record any damage to structures such as nerves or tendons, and at this stage *do not hesitate to seek help*. With a scalp laceration, make sure that you look at the epicranium for evidence of a skull fracture.

(5) Excise damaged, devitalized or dirty fat and muscle (Fig. 2.12). Fat which is loose, grey or covered with dirt is easily seen and should be cut back until it bleeds using either a scalpel or curved dissecting scissors. Take care not to cause further damage. Bruised or dead muscle is dusky and does not twitch when lightly grasped with a dissecting forceps. Again, cut it back until it bleeds.

Skin usually needs to be trimmed only to get rid of ragged edges to allow neat closure. Always check the viability of any flap that is less broad than it is long, particularly if its base is distal on a limb. The commonest example is a flap of skin detached on the anterior aspect of the tibia in an elderly lady who has fallen against a relatively

Fig. 2.11

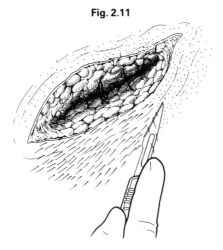

Fig. 2.12

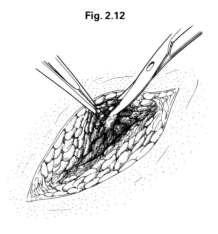

sharp edge – such as the step of a public transport vehicle. If the flap is dusky blue or if it fails to bleed when it is trimmed, then it is not viable and the skin must be cut back until free bleeding is obtained. Again, seek advice before trying to do anything clever to close such a defect.

(6) Secure haemostasis by grasping blood vessels (but as little surrounding tissue) with fine haemostats. Ligate with fine synthetic absorbable (3/0), or twist off as shown (Fig. 2.13).

(7) Close the wound with one or two layers. The latter is valuable:
   (i) to obliterate a dead space
   (ii) to unite a structural layer such as the epicranial aponeurosis in the scalp or the muscles of the face.
       The deep layer is best closed with the knot lying internally (Fig. 2.14). A synthetic absorbable should be used. In some circumstances, the deep layer can be placed so that it picks up the deep aspect of the dermis and so provides some support for the skin closure. If this is done, only tape is needed to close the skin (Fig. 2.15).

(8) For skin closure otherwise, use 4/0 nylon or polypropylene either as a simple over and over or as a vertical mattress suture (Figs. 2.14 and 2.16).

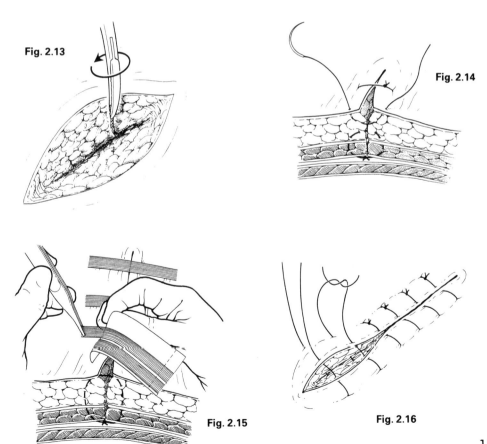

Fig. 2.13

Fig. 2.14

Fig. 2.15

Fig. 2.16

USING FINE SUTURES AND A NEEDLE HOLDER

Most of the simple suturing you will do is best undertaken with small, half-circle cutting needles on a needle holder. Eyeless needles should be used unless you are working in circumstances where their cost cannot be borne. The alternative technique is to use a three eighths circle needle held in the hand, but we do not recommend this.

(1) Lift and slightly evert the flap with a toothed dissecting forceps (Fig. 2.17).
(2) Hold the needle holder either with a standard grip through the rings, but preferably, and as you become more experienced, with a palm grip (Figs. 2.18A and B).
(3) Drive the needle initially vertically through the flap and then follow through with a circular motion (Fig. 2.19) while steadying the tissue with the dissecting forceps.
(4) Catch the needle tip with either the forceps or needle holder (Figs. 2.20A and B) and draw it through. If it is convenient, put the needle through both aspects of the wound with one movement, but when you are inexperienced it is usually easier to do one flap at a time.

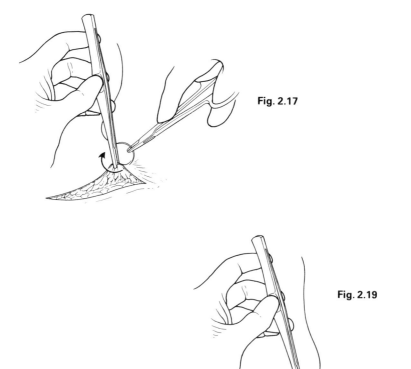

Fig. 2.17

Fig. 2.19

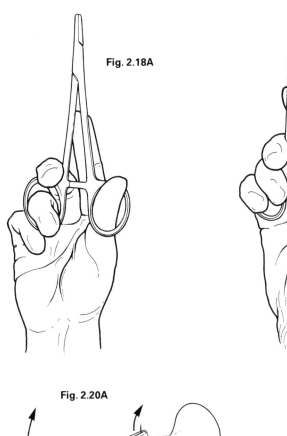

Fig. 2.18A

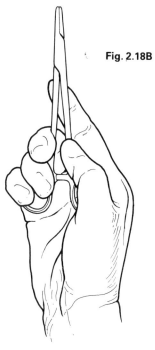

Fig. 2.18B

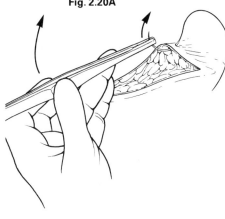

Fig. 2.20A

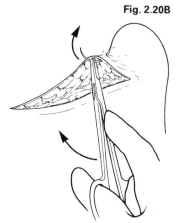

Fig. 2.20B

Chapter 3

Injections and anaesthesia

Injection techniques

The most common injection the doctor is called upon to give is by the intravenous route. However, from time to time, he or she may have to give an injection by the alternative routes. Before any injection, the hands should be washed and the area to be injected cleaned. Always double check the drug you are to administer, particularly if someone else has drawn it up for you.

SITES OF INJECTION

Intravenous

Intravenous injections are given using the same technique as for venesection (see p. 36). A tourniquet is placed around the upper arm and a suitable vein chosen in the antecubital fossa. Once the needle with a syringe containing the drug for administration has been inserted into the vein and blood withdrawn to confirm success, the tourniquet is released and the substance injected. The administration of large volumes of drugs, such as required in chemotherapy, is facilitated by the insertion of a 'butterfly' needle which can be temporarily secured in position with tape. Drugs which need to be given over a long time scale are best delivered through an intravenous infusion set after inserting an intravenous cannula (see p. 40).

After injections through a 'butterfly' cannula, the syringe and needle should be discarded and further injections given with a fresh needle and syringe. This removes the stage of re-sheathing needles for possible further use – a procedure which places the doctor at risk of an inoculation injury from the needle stick.

Intradermal

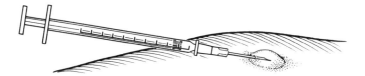

Fig. 3.1   The intradermal technique is mainly employed for the
administration of certain vaccines and for 'raising a weal' with local
anaesthetic agents (p. 25). Insert a 25G needle (orange in the UK) just into
the tough dermal layer at an oblique angle to the skin. Halt its forward
progress while it is still encountering resistance and inject the substance.

Subcutaneous

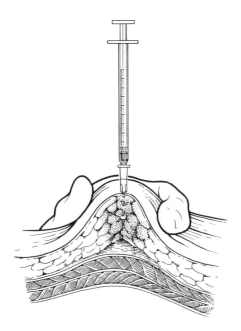

Fig. 3.2   The subcutaneous route is for the administration of local
anaesthesia, heparin and insulin. Insert a size 25G needle with the
appropriate syringe (usually 1 ml for injection of heparin and insulin) at
right angles into the skin of the lower abdomen or deltoid region. Pierce
the skin with the needle/syringe combination held like a dart so that rapid
and virtually painless penetration is made.

Intramuscular

This technique is usually used for intermittent administration of analgesia and antibiotics, as well as for some vaccines. Use a size 21G needle (green in the UK) for intramuscular injection into the buttock and thigh and a size 23G needle (blue in the UK) for intradeltoid injections.

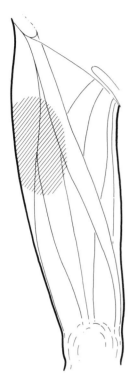

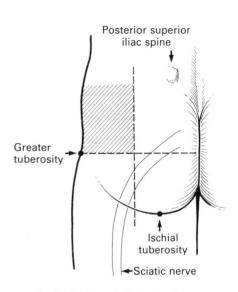

Fig. 3.3B *Buttock* — inject into the upper outer quadrant of the buttock.

Fig. 3.3A *Thigh* — inject into the muscular bulk of the quadriceps muscle on the anterolateral aspect one third of the way down from the hip.

Fig. 3.3C *Deltoid* — inject into the fleshy part of the deltoid muscle approximately 5 cm below the acromion. The procedure is facilitated by the patient placing his or her hand on the ipsilateral hip.

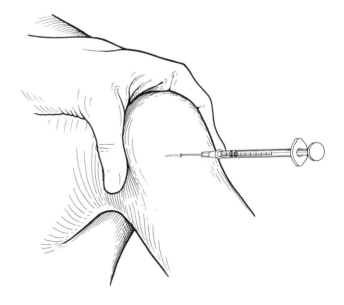

The principles of local anaesthesia will be described in detail here and thereafter only referred to in the text.

GENERAL POINTS

Local anaesthesia should not usually be used in inflamed or infected tissues as rapid systemic absorption may occur leading to toxic side effects. Absorption of the agent into the systemic circulation is responsible for the termination of action. Thus, decreasing local blood flow by vasoconstriction (using adrenaline) or applying a tourniquet will prolong the action.

CHOICE OF ANAESTHETIC

(1) *Lignocaine* is by far the most common agent used and is recommended for most minor procedures. It can be combined with adrenaline to reduce bleeding, as in operations on the face and scalp. It should *never* be used in surgery on extremities such as the ear, digits and penis as vasoconstriction can result in ischaemia.

Solutions: 0.5% (5 mg/ml)
1% (10 mg/ml)
2% (20 mg/ml)
with adrenaline 1:200 000 (500 μg/100 ml)
The maximum dose of lignocaine is 200 mg if used on its own, or 500 mg when combined with adrenaline. The maximum safe dose of adrenaline is 500 μg.
(2) *Bupivacaine* is used for prolonged anaesthesia as required in regional blocks, epidural blocks and spinal anaesthesia. Its action lasts up to 4–8 hours, and the maximum dose is 150 mg/4 hours.
(3) *Prilocaine* is short-acting, with a maximum dose of 400 mg when used alone or 600 mg when used with adrenaline.
N.B. These doses are based on a 70 kg adult.

TOXIC EFFECTS

If the maximum dose is exceeded or the agent allowed to escape into the general circulation, agitation, convulsions and cardiac arrhythmias (including cardiac arrest) can occur. When faced with a convulsion, 10–20 mg of intravenous diazepam should be administered in the first instance. If this fails to control the seizure, then 50–100 mg of chlorpromazine is given, also intravenously. Prolonged refractive generalized convulsions may require the administration of intravenous thiopentone for control.

ROUTES OF ADMINISTRATION

(1) Local infiltration
(2) Regional nerve block
(3) Epidural and spinal
(4) Bier's block
(5) Topical:
   Spray – used to anaesthetize the oropharynx and vocal cords before endotracheal intubation and gastroscopy
   Gel – used to anaesthetize the male urethra before catheterization
   Cream – applied to the mucous membrane of the mouth or to the skin before cannulation in children.

TECHNIQUES OF ADMINISTRATION

Infiltration for a straight line incision

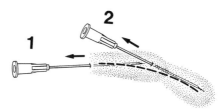

Fig. 3.4   Insert a 23G needle (blue in the UK) and syringe under the skin (in the subcutaneous tissues beneath the dermis) up to the hilt of the needle in the line of the incision. After drawing back to ensure that the needle is not in a vessel, inject local anaesthetic while withdrawing the needle and syringe. If one length of the needle does not cover the distance of the planned incision, re-insert the needle through the anaesthetized skin and repeat the process. If a large area of anaesthesia is required, change the blue needle for a larger one after the initial injection.

Infiltration for an elliptical incision

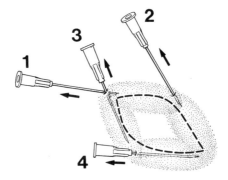

Fig. 3.5   Insert a 23G needle (blue) along each side of the planned ellipse and inject local anaesthetic on withdrawal. Re-insertion of the needle midway along the ellipse on each side allows the second half of the planned incision to be anaesthetized without injecting through unanaesthetized skin.

Infiltration of a wound

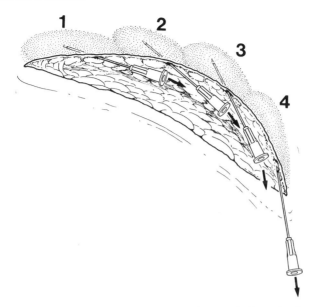

Fig. 3.6   After the wound edges have been thoroughly cleaned with a mild antiseptic such as Savlon (ICI), infiltrate the local anaesthetic into each side of the wound working from one end to the other. Always inject anaesthetic after full insertion of the needle and while it is being withdrawn. Before injection, take care to ensure that the needle is not in a vessel. If the wound is very contaminated, inject through the skin rather than the wound edges.

Raising a weal

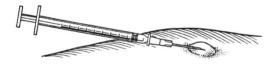

Fig. 3.7   Use a small 'insulin' syringe with a 25G needle (orange in the UK). Firmly enter the dermis with the needle/syringe combination at an oblique angle to the skin, to avoid going right through into the subcutaneous tissues. Apply firm pressure to the syringe to raise a circular weal 2–3 mm in diameter, which will turn white.

Regional anaesthesia

NERVE BLOCKS AT THE WRIST

It is possible to anaesthetize all three nerves serving the hand by infiltration at the wrist. Knowledge of the anatomical distribution of the nerves is essential so that the correct block is used for the procedure to be performed. Eliciting paraesthesia is a very useful sign that the needle is correctly sited; however, should it not occur then the anaesthetic solution should be injected in a fan-shaped distribution at the anatomical position of the nerve.

Equipment
(1) A 23G needle
(2) A 5 ml syringe
(3) 3–5 ml 1% lignocaine.

Complications
(1) Direct neural injection
(2) Vascular injection and injury with distal gangrene or necrosis.

Ulnar nerve block

Position

The arm is held abducted with the forearm supinated – the use of an arm board is helpful. The operator should sit on the ulnar side of the arm.

Anatomy

The ulnar nerve lies deep to the flexor carpi ulnaris (FCU) tendon at the wrist proximal to the pisiform bone.

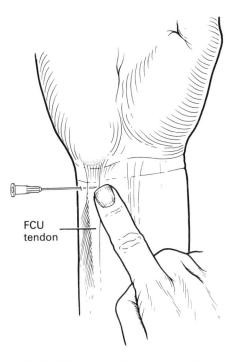

FCU
tendon

Fig. 3.8   Identify the FCU tendon at the proximal wrist crease by asking
the patient to flex the wrist against resistance. The site for insertion of the
needle is a point beneath the tendon on the ulnar border of the forearm
at the level of the proximal wrist crease. Insert the needle and syringe
towards the radial border of the wrist parallel to the floor for 1.0–1.5 cm.
During this, ask the patient when he feels a tingling sensation. When
paraesthesia is elicited, the needle should be withdrawn slightly and
3–5 ml of lignocaine are injected.

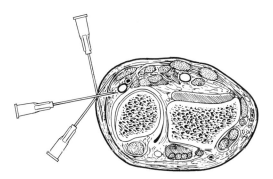

Fig. 3.9   Should total anaesthesia of the skin be necessary, give another
injection of lignocaine. First withdraw the needle to the subcutaneous
tissue, then insert it into this layer in a dorsal direction and inject lignocaine
along the outer border of the ulna. Subsequently, direct the needle
anterior to the FCU tendon and give a further injection of anaesthetic. This
blocks the palmar and dorsal cutaneous branches.

Median nerve block

Position

The arm is positioned as described for ulnar nerve block. The operator should sit on the ulnar side of the right arm and the radial side of the left arm.

Anatomy

The median nerve lies beneath the deep fascia between the tendons of palmaris longus (PL) and flexor carpi radialis (FCR) slightly under cover of the PL.

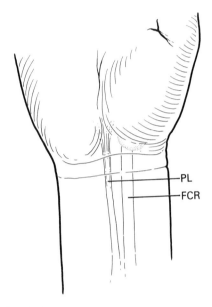

Fig. 3.10   Identify the PL and FCR tendons by resisted flexion. Mark the radial edge of the PL 2 cm proximal to the distal wrist crease; this is the point of insertion. If the PL is absent, mark the same point 1 cm medial to the edge of the FCR.

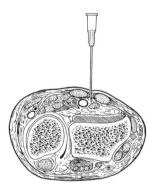

Fig. 3.11   Insert the needle perpendicular to the skin and advance 0.5–1.0 cm in depth until paraesthesia is felt (this is important as failure to elicit paraesthesia usually means that the needle is still above the deep fascia). Inject 3–5 ml of lignocaine at this point.

Radial nerve block

Position

The arm is rested on an arm board with the palm downward and the thumb extended. The operator sits on the radial side of the arm.

Anatomy

The cutaneous branches of the radial nerve run superficial to the extensor pollicis longus tendon (EPL), where they are easily palpable and alongside the extensor pollicis brevis tendon (EPB).

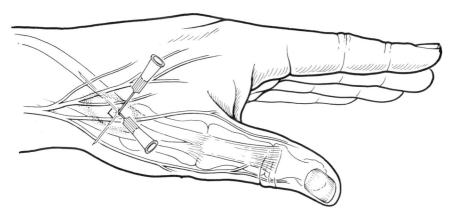

Fig. 3.12 Identify the anatomical snuffbox and the tendons of EPL and EPB by extending the thumb. Mark the tendons. Palpate the base of the first metacarpal – this is the site for insertion of the needle. Insert the needle along the line of the EPL tendon towards the wrist in the subcutaneous plane. Inject 2–3 ml of anaesthetic as the needle is withdrawn. Redirect the needle from the point of insertion at 90° to the line of the EPB tendon. Inject 1–2 ml of lignocaine as the needle is withdrawn.

DIGITAL NERVE BLOCKADE

The injection of digital nerves at the base of a finger is a commonly used technique. However, it is potentially the most hazardous method of anaesthetizing the finger because of the potential for ischaemia and necrosis. The technique of blockade of the nerves in the metacarpal spaces is safer. Vasoconstrictors must NEVER be used with either method.

Metacarpal block

Position

The hand is laid flat with the palm down and the fingers spread apart.

Anatomy

The palmar digital nerve runs dorsal to the superficial palmar ligament in a neurovascular bundle.

Digital block at the base of the finger

Position

The hand is laid flat with the palm down and the fingers spread slightly apart.

Anatomy

At the base of the finger, the volar digital nerves run in a neurovascular bundle alongside the flexor sheaths. The smaller dorsal digital nerves run on the dorsolateral aspect of the finger.

Beware
(1) The swollen injured finger
(2) Patients with peripheral arterial disease or Raynaud's phenomenon
(3) Never use vasoconstrictors
(4) Never use more than 2 ml on each side of the finger
(5) The tourniquet time should be 15 minutes maximum.

Complications

Vascular injury or injection leading to digital gangrene and necrosis.

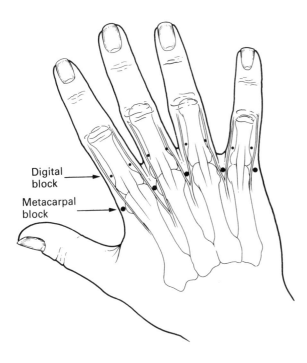

Digital block

Metacarpal block

Fig. 3.13   Insert the needle directly between the metacarpal heads for a metacarpal block and at the base of the finger alongside the proximal phalanx for digital block.

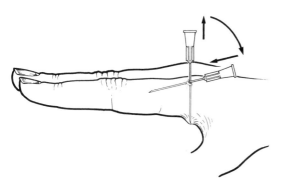

Fig. 3.14   Metacarpal block. Advance the needle perpendicularly until the skin on the palm is tented slightly; this can be felt by placing a finger beneath the palm. Withdraw the needle 5 mm and inject 2–3 ml of lignocaine. Should it be necessary to anaesthetize the dorsal branches, direct the needle as it is withdrawn towards the dorsal nerves at the base of the proximal phalanx. This procedure is performed on either side of the finger to be anaesthetized.

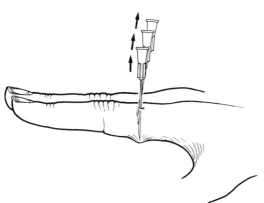

Fig. 3.15   Digital block. Advance the needle until the palmar surface is tented, as felt with a finger beneath the path of the needle. Withdraw the needle 2–3 mm and inject 1 ml of anaesthetic. Then withdraw the needle almost out of the skin and inject a further 0.5 ml. Repeat this on the other side of the finger.

31

AXILLARY NERVE BLOCK

This technique enables procedures to be carried out on the arm including minor surgery and manipulation of fractures. By anaesthetizing the upper arm, it allows the application of a tourniquet without causing the discomfort often associated with their use.

Position

The patient is supine with the arm held abducted to 90°. If possible, resting the hand behind the head is helpful.

Equipment

(1) A 21G needle
(2) A 50 ml syringe with 10 cm of extension tubing
(3) 40 ml of 1% lignocaine with 1:200 000 adrenaline (for a 70 kg man), see p. 23
(4) A tourniquet
(5) An 18G intravenous cannula.

Special points

(1) The patient must be starved.
(2) Intravenous access must be obtained in the opposite hand before undertaking this procedure.
(3) Axillary block must not be done in the presence of either infection or malignancy.
(4) Analgesia takes 25–30 minutes to develop following injection. A further indication of successful block is the sympathetic block that occurs, with the arm becoming warm and dry.

Complications

(1) Intravascular injection
(2) Neural injury

Fig 3.16

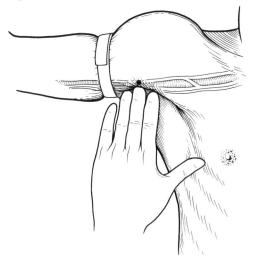

Fig. 3.16   The axillary artery and the cords of the brachial plexus which surround the artery are enclosed in a strong fascial sheath into which the injection must be given. With the arm abducted, palpate the axillary artery against the upper humerus and make a mark over the most proximal point at which it can be felt in the axilla. Anaesthetize the skin at this point. Apply a tourniquet just distal to the injection point and keep it on for 10 minutes following injection of the analgesic agent to ensure blockade of the musculocutaneous nerve.

Fig. 3.17A   Insert the needle through the marked point and direct it superior to the artery. You will feel a 'give' on going through the axillary fascia (this feeling of entering the sheath is helped if you blunt the needle slightly before starting). The needle may show transmitted pulsation and paraesthesia may be elicited, both indicating that the needle tip is correctly sited (Fig. 3.17B). Connect the syringe via the extension tubing and aspirate to ensure that the needle is not in the artery; then inject the analgesic solution (see p. 23 for volumes and concentrations). An alternative method is to inject both inferior and superior to the artery.

Fig. 3.18   On withdrawal, inject 2–3 ml of analgesic solution subcutaneously along a line 90° to the long axis of the arm on both sides of the injection point to block the intercostobrachial nerve; this prevents any discomfort from a tourniquet applied to the upper arm.

Fig. 3.17A

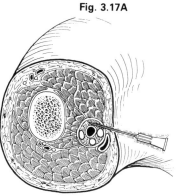

Fig. 3.18

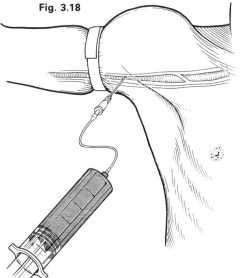

Fig. 3.17B

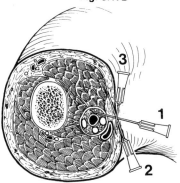

Vascular access

Venepuncture

This is a basic procedure for obtaining blood samples. The femoral vein should be used only when it is impossible to obtain blood from any vein in either arm.

Position

The patient should be supine with the arm to be punctured resting comfortably by the side. For femoral puncture, the groin should be exposed with the leg extended and slightly abducted.

Equipment

(1) A 21G needle
(2) A syringe (size according to the amount required)
(3) Specimen bottles
(4) A tourniquet or blood pressure cuff.

Special points

Do not allow the patient to flex the elbow after removing the needle as haematoma is more likely to occur from that manoeuvre. The risk of a needle stick injury is reduced if the used needles are immediately discarded without re-sheathing.

Complications

(1) Injury to local structures
(2) Haematoma formation
(3) Thrombosis

ANTECUBITAL VEIN PUNCTURE

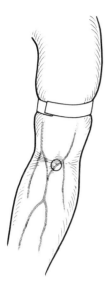

Fig. 4.1 Apply the tourniquet to the upper arm and identify an appropriate superficial vein both visually and by palpation. Clean the skin and raise a bleb of local anaesthetic if the patient is apprehensive.

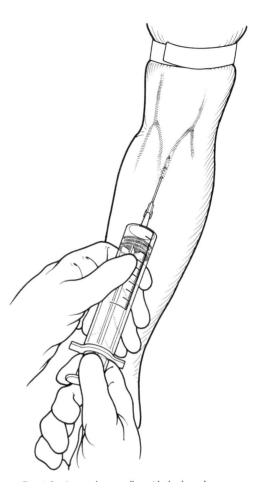

Fig. 4.3 Insert the needle, with the bevel upwards, through the skin beside the vein and then bring the point over the vein and puncture this with a second movement. If the skin is thin, both movements can be combined with practice and a relaxed patient. Use the left hand now to steady the syringe and the right to withdraw the blood required. Release the tourniquet and, in one movement, press the alcohol wipe or a cotton wool ball against the puncture site and withdraw the needle. Pressure is necessary for about 30 seconds to prevent bleeding. Cover the puncture site with a small plaster.

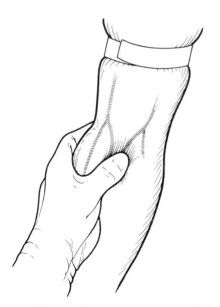

Fig. 4.2 With the thumb of the left hand, tense the skin at the elbow by gentle traction.

FEMORAL VEIN PUNCTURE

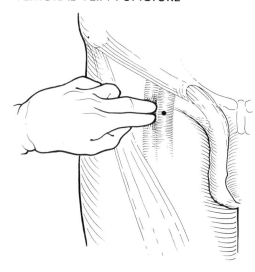

Fig. 4.4   Identify the position of the femoral vein 2 cm below the inguinal ligament by palpation of the femoral artery which lies immediately lateral to the vein. Clean the skin and raise a bleb of local anaesthetic if the patient is apprehensive.

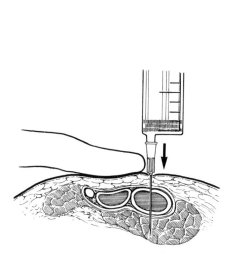

Fig. 4.5   With the left middle finger on the femoral pulse, insert the needle to the hilt at a right angle to the skin at the tip of this finger.

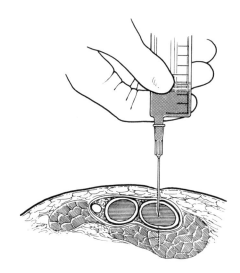

Fig. 4.6   With the left hand holding the syringe and the right gently pulling back on the plunger, withdraw the needle slowly until blood flows freely into the syringe. When aspirating, it is very important to hold the syringe steady as it can easily slip out of the vein. Withdraw the needle and syringe and apply pressure to the site of puncture for two minutes. Cover the site with a plaster.

CAPILLARY BLOOD SAMPLE

A common technique for obtaining blood samples in the neonate is to remove blood from the heel. Capillary samples can also be taken from the fleshy part of the thumb in the adult, most commonly for measurement of blood glucose. The 'heel prick' technique in the neonate is described here.

Equipment
(1) A lance
(2) Capillary tubes
(3) Plasticine
(4) Petroleum jelly.

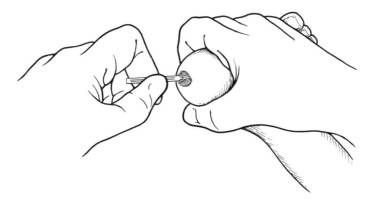

Fig. 4.7   Grasp the baby's heel in the palm of the hand with the ankle. After cleaning the skin, apply vaseline and plunge a lance into the bulging flesh.

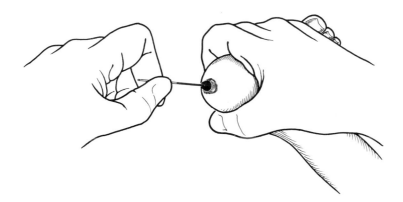

Fig. 4.8   The vaseline allows a globule of blood to form at the site of the injury; collect this in a capillary tube, as illustrated. Seal the sample by inserting the end of the capillary tube in plasticine.

Setting up an intravenous infusion

This is a standard technique for the administration of iso-osmotic fluids. Cannulae should be changed at intervals no longer than 72 hours.

Position

The patient should be supine with the arm to be cannulated by their side. A waterproof sheet underneath saves the sheets from blood – and you from the nurses' wrath.

Equipment

(1) An intravenous cannula 14–22G. The faster the infusion rate needs to be, the larger the size of cannula required; for standard replacement, an 18G cannula is adequate. For blood transfusion, a size 16G or 14G is necessary.
(2) Intravenous fluid with a giving set primed and ready for connection
(3) Adhesive tape cut to length
(4) Local anaesthetic drawn up into an insulin syringe
(5) A three-way tap if more than one infusion, or drugs, are to be given.

Special points

If at any stage it becomes apparent that the cannula is not in the vein, then start afresh elsewhere. It is not acceptable to attempt to reinsert the metal needle into the cannula as the plastic may be cut and there is a danger of embolization. In children it is advisable to apply local anaesthetic cream to potential sites of cannulation 60 minutes before.

Complications

(1) Failure to cannulate
(2) Extraluminal infusion. It is sensible, if in doubt, to aspirate before starting the infusion; this is particularly so if irritant fluids are being given
(3) Superficial phlebitis, which may become a cellulitis
(4) Thrombosis
(5) 'Tissued cannula' where the tip has eroded the wall of the vein and the infusion is running into the subcutaneous tissues.

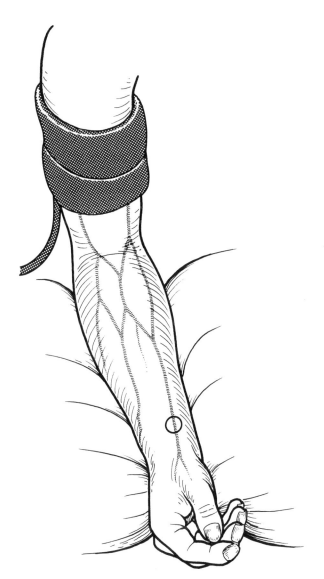

Fig. 4.9   To select a vein, inflate a BP cuff to just below diastolic pressure
on the upper arm. Use a vein on the dorsum of the forearm if possible.
Avoid the antecubital fossa, unless there is great urgency, and do not use
the hand; both of these are uncomfortable for the patient. Shave a hirsute
arm. Raise a bleb of local anaesthetic at the site of entry.

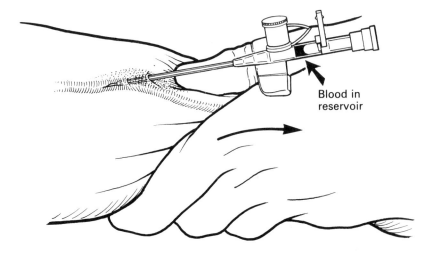

Blood in
reservoir

Fig. 4.10   Stretch the skin over the vein by applying traction with the left
hand. Insert the cannula through the skin and, with a second movement,
into the vein. A flashback of blood indicates that the vein has been
punctured. Advance the needle 3–5 mm further to ensure that the plastic
cannula is also within the lumen of the vein. Make sure that when inserting
the cannula through the skin the needle does not back out of the cannula.

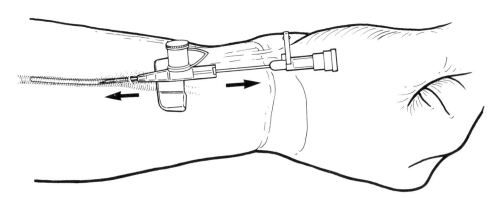

Fig. 4.11   Withdraw the needle slightly and slide the cannula over the
needle into the vein up to the hub. Release the tourniquet.

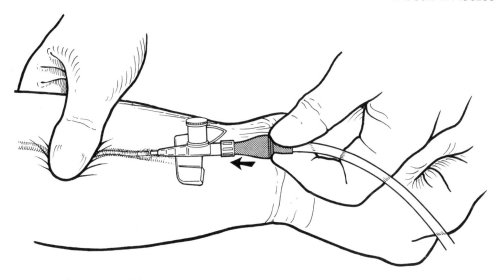

Fig. 4.12   Withdraw the needle while applying pressure over the vein just proximal to the tip of the cannula. Attach the giving set with a luer lock fitting.

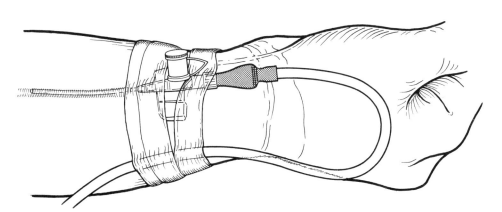

Fig. 4.13   Secure the cannula and giving set in place with the tape. A splint may be necessary if the cannula crosses a joint.

Cut-down for venous access

When an intravenous infusion is to be set up, either as an emergency or electively, venous access by direct puncture can be difficult and a cut-down needed. This most commonly occurs in small children and obese adults. For resuscitation in an emergency, a central line is most appropriate (see p. 46). The antecubital fossa is the best area for exposing a large vein and if this fails, the saphenofemoral junction should be exposed and the long saphenous vein cannulated. A quick slash at this site can be life-saving as many a surgeon can attest. The lower leg should not be used as this is a low flow area with a serious risk of gangrene, particularly in children.

Position
The patient should be supine with the antecubital fossa exposed.

Equipment
(1) Self-retaining retractor (if available)
(2) A scalpel and a size 10 blade
(3) Curved dissecting scissors (McIndoe)
(4) Non-toothed dissecting forceps
(5) An intravenous cannula (size 16G or larger)
(6) 3/0 suture material, preferably absorbable.
(7) If the patient is conscious, local anaesthetic should be used.

Complications
(1) Local skin ulceration and infection
(2) Superficial thrombophlebitis.

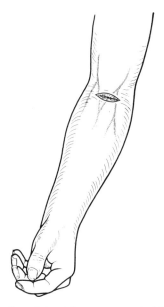

Fig. 4.14   Make a transverse incision across the middle of the antecubital fossa and extend it down through the superficial fat.

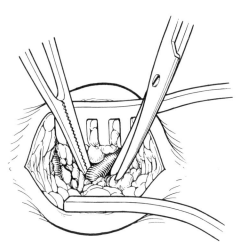

Fig. 4.15   After the self-retaining retractor has been inserted, explore the fat with gentle dissection for the large veins. Once found, clear the vein of surrounding tissue for 1 cm and pass a suture around it both proximally and distally; tie the latter.

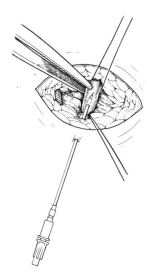

Fig. 4.16   Introduce the cannula through the distal skin flap and pick up the vein with non-toothed forceps. If the vein is large, insert the cannula directly by direct puncture and, once in the vein, withdraw the needle. If the vein is small, nick it with scissors and extend the venotomy down one side by inserting one blade of the scissors; then insert the cannula without the needle.

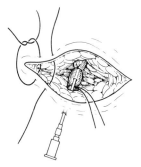

Fig. 4.17   Now tie the proximal suture to secure the cannula in the vein, and close the skin with interrupted 3/0 nylon sutures. It is prudent to stitch the cannula to the skin before dressing the wound.

Central vein cannulation

SELDINGER TECHNIQUE FOR VASCULAR CANNULATION

This technique for vascular access was described in 1953. The method can be used for both arterial and venous cannulation.

Position

The position of the patient will be according to the procedure to be performed.

Equipment

The equipment necessary is often found in a variety of pre-packed kits.

(1) A needle and cannula
(2) Spring-coiled guide wire
(3) A vascular catheter
(4) A three-way tap
(5) A scalpel with size 15 blade
(6) A prepared intravenous infusion.

Complications

(1) Haematoma
(2) Injury to local structures
(3) Thrombosis
(4) Infection.

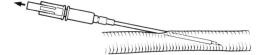

Fig. 4.18   Perform vessel puncture in the standard manner for the particular vessel; always use a syringe on the end of the needle so that you can aspirate blood to ensure correct positioning of the needle tip. A nick through the skin with a scalpel blade is helpful.

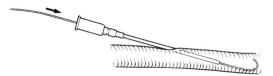

Fig. 4.19   This step will vary according to the kit being used. Introduce the guide wire into the vessel, either directly through the needle or through an introducer cannula. The latter involves threading the introducer cannula over the needle into the vein, as for a peripheral venous cannulation. Then remove the needle leaving just the introducer cannula in the lumen of the vessel.

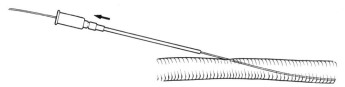

Fig. 4.20   Once the guide wire is in place, remove the needle or cannula; when doing this, however, take care to fix the guide wire to prevent accidental removal.

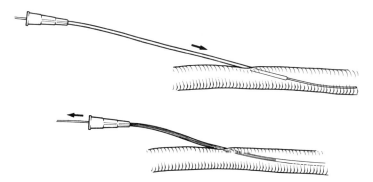

Fig. 4.21   With the guide wire in situ, pass the definitive catheter over the guide wire into the vessel. When this has been placed in the desired position, remove the guide wire – again, holding the catheter to prevent its accidental removal. (A tissue dilator is sometimes provided for use before passing the definitive catheter). Finally, connect the infusion or monitoring device.

47

SUBCLAVIAN VEIN CANNULATION

The infraclavicular approach to the subclavian vein provides a suitable route for central vein cannulation, although it does carry the risk of pneumothorax.

Position

The patient is supine with the bed tilted 5–10°, head down. A sand-bag or pillow is placed between the shoulder blades to throw the shoulders and head back. The head is turned towards the opposite side.

Equipment

(1) A central venous catheter, which will be either a long version of a standard peripheral intravenous cannula or a catheter requiring a Seldinger technique for placement. The former is preferable in an emergency.
(2) Local anaesthetic
(3) A size 15 scalpel blade
(4) An intravenous infusion ready to connect
(5) Nylon suture 3/0.

Management

(1) Following insertion take a chest x-ray to check the position of the catheter and to exclude a pneumothorax.
(2) An aseptic technique whenever giving sets are changed.

Complications

(1) Pneumothorax
(2) Haemothorax
(3) Arterial puncture
(4) Air embolism
(5) Central line infection
(6) Central vein thrombosis.

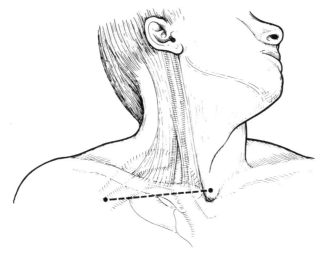

Fig. 4.22   Identify the midpoint of the clavicle – this should be where the clavicle curves posteriorly towards the acromioclavicular joint. Make a mark 1–2 cm below the lower border of the bone at this point. Infiltrate local anaesthetic at the site of the incision.

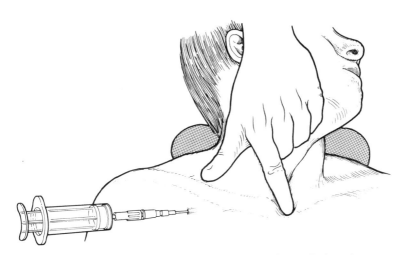

Fig. 4.23   Make a small nick through the skin. Push the needle through the skin aiming towards the suprasternal notch. Gently advance the needle until it abuts against the lower border of the clavicle. Angle the needle slightly and advance it beneath the lower border of the bone, still aiming at the suprasternal notch; aspirate gently while advancing. The needle should run parallel to the floor approximately 15° headwards, although it may be necessary to angle the needle superiorly initially to ensure that contact is made with the lower border of the clavicle. When blood is aspirated, advance the needle a few millimetres further to ensure that the outer cannula is within the lumen of the vein, and then slide the catheter over the needle into the vein. Withdraw the needle and immediately connect the infusion to prevent any risk of air embolism. Fix the cannula securely in place; a suture around the cannula is a good method.

49

INTERNAL JUGULAR VEIN CANNULATION

There are several approaches to the internal jugular vein – we have chosen to describe two of the more common ones. Internal jugular vein cannulation is performed on many thousands of patients each year by anaesthetists and it is sensible to learn this technique in theatre under their guidance before attempting it on the ward.

Position

The patient is supine with a head down tilt of 30–45° if tolerable. The head is rested on the bed (any pillows are removed) and turned to the opposite side as far as possible. It is frequently possible to see the pulsation of the jugular vein, and this can act as a guide to the line of insertion.

Equipment

(1) A central venous catheter (it is best to use a 14G needle and cannulae are generally less flexible and easier to manipulate)
(2) Local anaesthetic
(3) An intravenous infusion ready to connect
(4) Nylon suture 3/0.

Management

(1) Rigorous asepsis when changing infusions, because the wound in the neck and the intravenous connections are all potential sources of infection.
(2) A chest x-ray, to check the position and for a pneumothorax.

Special points

(1) The needle should not be advanced further than 5 cm into the neck.
(2) Should there be difficulty in aspirating after advancing the cannula into the vein, withdraw while aspirating and, when there is free flow back into the syringe, flush the cannula with the blood and advance again while flushing. This will straighten out any kinks in the cannula.
(3) The low approach to the vein is sometimes easier if the landmarks are easy to identify; however, it is more hazardous than the high approach.
(4) If the carotid artery is punctured by mistake, the needle and cannula should be removed. This does not preclude a further attempt at venous cannulation on the same side.

Complications

(1) Central vein thrombosis
(2) Central line sepsis
(3) Pneumothorax
(4) Injury to local structures
(5) Haematoma.

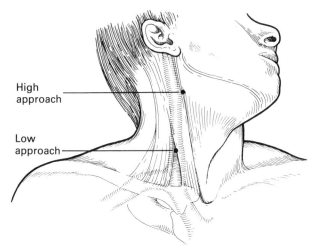

Fig. 4.24   For the high approach, identify the midpoint of a line drawn between the sternal notch and mastoid; this is the site of insertion. For the low approach, identify the apex of the triangle formed by the sternal and clavicular heads of the sternomastoid and the clavicle inferiorly. The venous pulsation is often visible to guide your line of insertion.

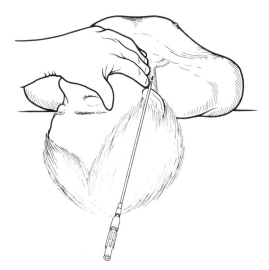

Fig. 4.25   For the high approach, place the tips of all four fingers along the carotid artery; this identifies the line of the internal jugular vein which lies lateral to it. The line of insertion should be towards the nipple and it will usually take the needle through a part of the sternomastoid muscle. Introduce the needle and cannula, through a stab incision made with a no. 11 scalpel blade tip, with the right hand. Having decided on the correct line, use the left hand to steady the needle while advancing it with short stabbing movements, with the right hand aspirating at each advancement. The angle of the needle should be 15–20° downward at maximum – a common error is to go too deeply into the neck. When the vein is entered, rotate the whole needle and syringe by 180°. Check that blood can be freely aspirated. At this point, use the right hand to hold the needle steady, and the left hand to advance the cannula, with a twisting motion, up to its hub. Should there be any resistance at this point, it is worth trying to change the angle of the entire apparatus so that it is facing more medially. Connect the infusion and secure the cannula and tubing.
    For the low approach, use a similar method of advancement and aspiration. The direction is towards the nipple but at a steeper angle of 20–30°. The vein lies fairly superficially at this level and you should not advance the needle more than 2 cm in depth. A common error is to direct the needle too laterally.

CENTRAL VENOUS CATHETERIZATION WITH A DRUM CATHETER

This method is used for placement of a central venous line via a peripheral vein. It avoids the hazards of direct central vein catheterization (p. 48).

Position

The patient is supine with the arm resting comfortably by the side.

Equipment

(1) A basic dressing set
(2) A drum catheter cartridge
(3) An intravenous infusion prepared for connection.

Management

Check the position of the catheter tip with a chest x-ray. Should the catheter be in a neck vessel, it must be withdrawn until it lies at the level of the root of the neck. The catheter must *never* be withdrawn and then reinserted.

Complications

(1) Haematoma at the site of insertion
(2) Phlebitis at the site of insertion
(3) Central venous infection
(4) Central vein thrombosis
(5) Malposition of the catheter.

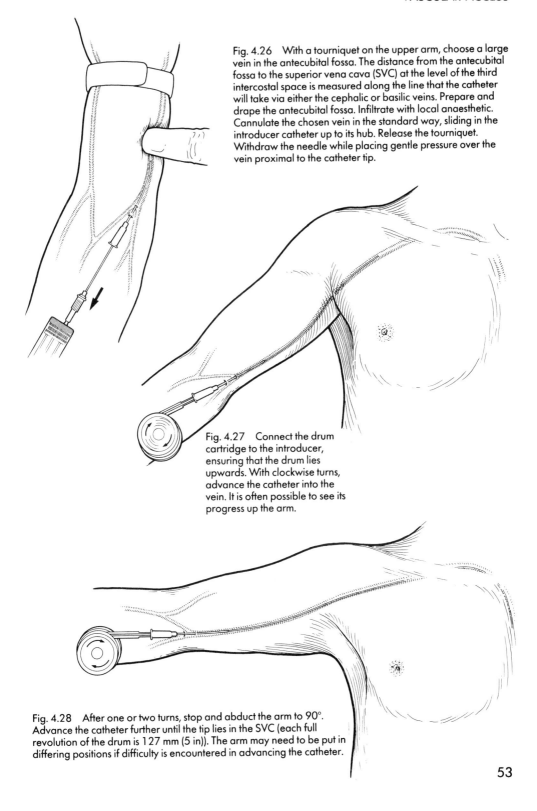

Fig. 4.26   With a tourniquet on the upper arm, choose a large vein in the antecubital fossa. The distance from the antecubital fossa to the superior vena cava (SVC) at the level of the third intercostal space is measured along the line that the catheter will take via either the cephalic or basilic veins. Prepare and drape the antecubital fossa. Infiltrate with local anaesthetic. Cannulate the chosen vein in the standard way, sliding in the introducer catheter up to its hub. Release the tourniquet. Withdraw the needle while placing gentle pressure over the vein proximal to the catheter tip.

Fig. 4.27   Connect the drum cartridge to the introducer, ensuring that the drum lies upwards. With clockwise turns, advance the catheter into the vein. It is often possible to see its progress up the arm.

Fig. 4.28   After one or two turns, stop and abduct the arm to 90°. Advance the catheter further until the tip lies in the SVC (each full revolution of the drum is 127 mm (5 in)). The arm may need to be put in differing positions if difficulty is encountered in advancing the catheter.

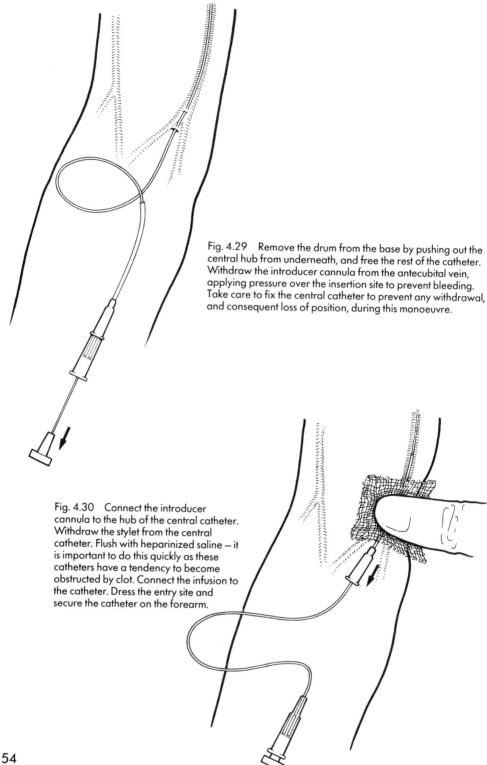

Fig. 4.29 Remove the drum from the base by pushing out the central hub from underneath, and free the rest of the catheter. Withdraw the introducer cannula from the antecubital vein, applying pressure over the insertion site to prevent bleeding. Take care to fix the central catheter to prevent any withdrawal, and consequent loss of position, during this manoeuvre.

Fig. 4.30 Connect the introducer cannula to the hub of the central catheter. Withdraw the stylet from the central catheter. Flush with heparinized saline — it is important to do this quickly as these catheters have a tendency to become obstructed by clot. Connect the infusion to the catheter. Dress the entry site and secure the catheter on the forearm.

CENTRAL VENOUS PRESSURE MEASUREMENT

In most instances, a central venous line is put in for the measurement of central venous pressure as an adjunct to monitoring fluid balance in the seriously ill patient. To do this, a manometer is connected to the system.

Position

The patient can be supine or semi-recumbent. The most important point is to ensure that the measurement is taken with the patient in the same position each time, and that the zero mark is the same each time.

Equipment
(1) A three-way tap
(2) Manometer tubing with centimetre markings
(3) A drip stand
(4) An indelible marker
(5) Extension intravenous tubing.

Special points

There are special attachments which can be used for fixing the manometer to drip stands. These are already marked and the tubing is clipped into place. A telescopic spirit level forms part of this equipment to ensure that the two zeros are at the same height.

Complications
(1) Misinformation because of failure to position the patient, the catheter and the measuring equipment accurately
(2) Air embolism while setting up the equipment
(3) The complications of central venous catheters.

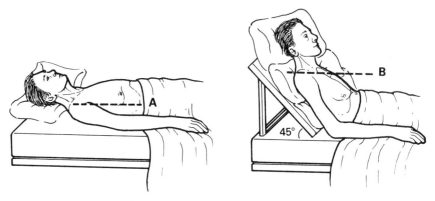

Fig. 4.31 With the patient supine, make a mark in the mid-axillary line at the level of the nipple (A). This point will be arbitrarily called zero as it indicates the level of the right atrium, the normal pressure of which is 0–5 mmHg. If the patient is sitting at 45°, the zero may be taken as the manubriosternal joint (B).

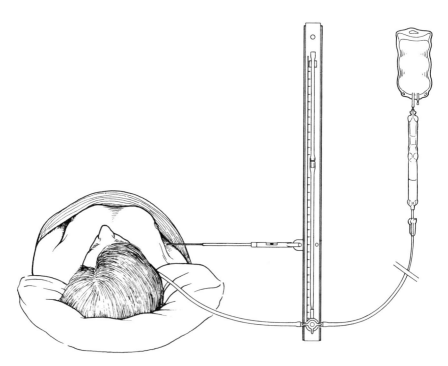

Fig. 4.32 Flush and lock the central venous catheter. Connect the intravenous infusion, manometer tubing and extension tubing to the three-way tap and flush through the extension tubing. Reconnect to the venous catheter with the infusion being run as before. Fix the graduated manometer tubing to the drip stand with tape. Zero is best taken at 10 cm so that a negative reading will register, as most tubing does not mark below zero. The zero mark on the patient and the zero mark on the tubing must be at the same level (see note on previous page).

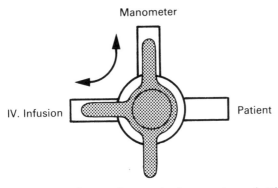

Manometer

IV. Infusion

Patient

Fig. 4.33   To take a reading, turn the three-way tap so that the manometer tubing is filled — to near the top — from the intravenous infusion.

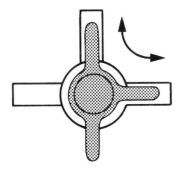

Fig. 4.34   Turn the tap so that the manometer tubing and venous catheter are in continuity. The fluid level in the manometer tubing will fall until a steady state is achieved; then take the reading in centimetres of water (the fluid level should swing with respiration).

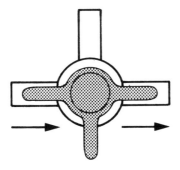

Fig. 4.35   Once the reading is done, turn the tap to continue the infusion until the next reading.

Arterial puncture

Arterial puncture is for the measurement of blood gases and pH.

Position

(1) *Radial artery*: The patient is supine and the arm lies by the side. An assistant holds the wrist and thumb extended. A rolled towel behind the wrist can be helpful.
(2) *Femoral artery*: The patient is supine with the groin exposed and the leg extended and slightly abducted.

Equipment

(1) A 23G butterfly needle for radial artery puncture; a 23G needle for femoral artery puncture
(2) A heparinized 2 ml syringe. Draw up 1 ml of 1000 U/ml heparin into the syringe. Squirt most of this away to leave a very small quantity at the tip. Ensure that there is no air in the syringe.
(3) A syringe cap
(4) Ice.

Special points

(1) When the needle is withdrawn, pressure is applied over the puncture site for 5 minutes.
(2) The syringe is capped following withdrawal and placed in a bag containing ice for transport to the laboratory.

Complications

(1) Thrombosis
(2) Embolism
(3) Spasm
(4) Gangrene
(5) Haematoma
(6) Infection
(7) Arteriovenous fistula formation
(8) Aneurysm formation.

Radial artery puncture

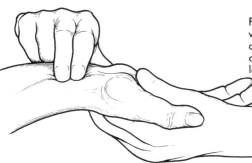

Fig. 4.36 Palpate the radial artery proximal to the wrist joint. Choose as the site of puncture a point approximately 1 cm proximal to the distal wrist crease, where the artery is easily felt. Raise a bleb of local anaesthetic at the proposed site of entry.

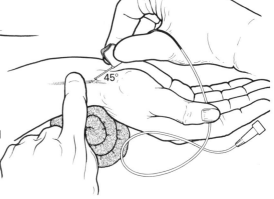

Fig. 4.37 Insert the butterfly needle through the skin at an angle of 45°. Advance the needle slowly at 45° with the index finger of the left hand feeling the radial pulse just proximally to give a guide to direction. The free flow of blood into the butterfly tubing indicates successful puncture. Connect the syringe to the butterfly and take the necessary amount of blood. Care is necessary to avoid any air in the system.

Femoral artery puncture

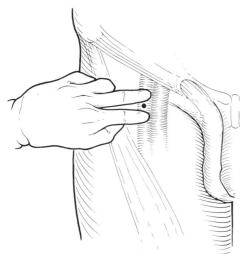

Fig. 4.38 Palpate the femoral artery 2 cm below the inguinal ligament at the mid-inguinal point which is halfway between the anterior superior iliac spine and the symphysis pubis. The site of puncture is directly over the artery where it is easily palpable between two fingers. Raise a bleb of local anaesthetic. Fix the artery between the middle and index fingers of the left hand.

Fig. 4.39 Insert the heparinized needle and syringe through the skin at right angles. Advance the needle slowly until there is free flow into the syringe, indicating successful puncture. Should there be any doubt as to whether it is arterial or venous blood, removing the syringe from the needle will demonstrate pulsatile flow if it is in the artery.

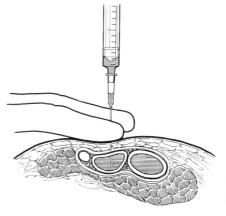

Arterial cannulation

Arterial cannulation is for pressure monitoring and/or frequent blood gas analysis. The radial artery is most commonly used.

Position

The patient is positioned as described for radial artery puncture.
For dorsalis pedis puncture, the foot is held slightly plantar flexed. The artery lies lateral to the extensor hallucis tendon and is crossed by the tendon of extensor hallucis brevis.

Equipment

(1) A 20G arterial cannula (it can be a venous catheter)
(2) Heparinized saline, 500 U in 500 ml
(3) A continuous flushing system with a rapid flush capability
(4) A three-way tap
(5) Extension tubing
(6) Adhesive tape.

Special points

(1) Before cannulation, Allen's test must be carried out to ensure adequate arterial circulation to the hand by the ulnar artery.
(2) A modified Seldinger type technique is possible using a catheterization set which has an integral guide wire system. Here, the artery is cannulated and a guide wire advanced into the lumen; the cannula is then advanced over the guide wire.
(3) The technique for dorsalis pedis cannulation is the same as for the radial artery.

Complications

Complications are as described for arterial puncture.

RADIAL ARTERY CANNULATION

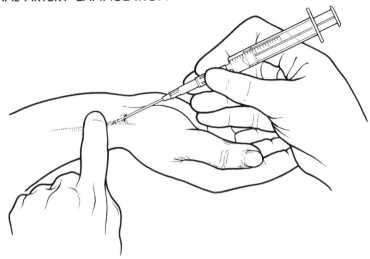

Fig. 4.40 The technique is the same as for arterial puncture except that the skin should be incised with a blade. When the artery is punctured with the needle, as indicated by a flashback, advance the plastic cannula over the needle to its hilt. It is sensible to ensure free arterial flow by aspiration before advancing the plastic cannula because the needle commonly penetrates the posterior wall of the artery. If aspiration is not successful, the needle is withdrawn until free flow occurs.

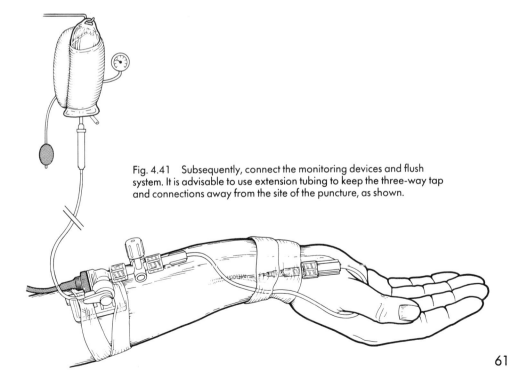

Fig. 4.41 Subsequently, connect the monitoring devices and flush system. It is advisable to use extension tubing to keep the three-way tap and connections away from the site of the puncture, as shown.

Chapter
5

Resuscitation

Basic cardiopulmonary resuscitation

airway

↓

breathing

↓

circulation

Every doctor should be capable of maintaining adequate oxygenation of the brain by mechanical means. It is an individual's responsibility to ensure that he or she knows the methods by which this is achieved and some of the therapeutic manoeuvres to restore cardiac rhythm. Practice with dummies is useful, as is taking any opportunity to practise endotracheal intubation under the supervision of an anaesthetist. Sadly, it is all too frequent to see medical staff at a loss about basic resuscitation or, when attempting it, doing it wrongly.

Position

For full cardiopulmonary resuscitation (CPR), the patient should be placed on his or her back on a firm surface.

Assessment

(1) Look for chest movement.
(2) Listen and feel for air movement.
(3) Feel for carotid or femoral pulses.

Special points

(1) One of the problems with aided ventilation by mechanical means is gaseous distension of the stomach. The Sellick manoeuvre of pressure over the cricoid, compressing the oesophagus between larynx and vertebra, will help prevent passive regurgitation as well as gastric inflation (see p. 88). The manoeuvre requires an assistant. It must not be performed during active vomiting.
(2) When 'a crash trolley' arrives, the airway can be protected by endotracheal intubation (see p. 80) or by placing an airway into the patient's mouth and using an Ambu bag, which can be attached to the oxygen supply for ventilation. Again, attention must be paid to adequate air movement by observation of the chest and by listening over both lung fields with a stethoscope. Suction facilities should be available on a crash trolley and used to clear the mouth and pharynx of secretions; this is essential before attempting intubation. It is important to give several good inflations with the Ambu bag before attempting endotracheal intubation. If intubation fails, go back to the Ambu bag and await the arrival of more experienced medical staff. Do not persist in repeated and ever more desperate attempts to intubate.

AIRWAY

Maintaining an airway

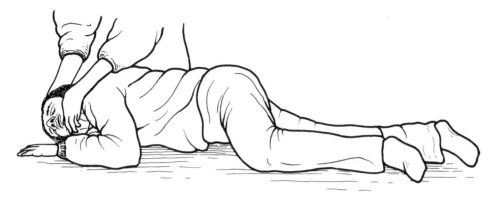

Fig. 5.1   If the person is breathing, place them in the recovery position.

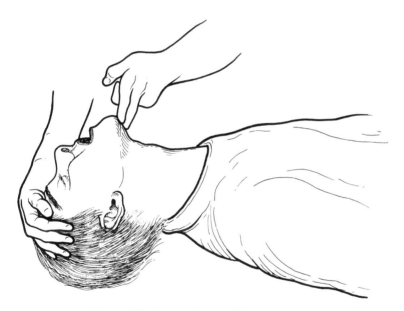

Fig. 5.2   If there is difficulty in or absence of breathing, an airway must be established. First, lift the tongue away from the posterior pharynx. Use the fingers of the left hand to hold the chin forwards and upwards whilst extending the neck slightly with the right hand. By placing the edge of your hand on the forehead it is possible to maintain the extended position at the same time as pinching the nose tight. If obstruction is caused by an object in the major airways, sweep a finger round the mouth first and follow by firm blows to the back. The use of the Heimlich manoeuvre may also be helpful (see p. 77). Should the obstruction remain and laryngoscopy with suction not be to hand, an urgent laryngotomy will be necessary (see p. 86). In the absence of breathing, mouth-to-mouth resuscitation is required.

BREATHING
Mouth-to-mouth resuscitation

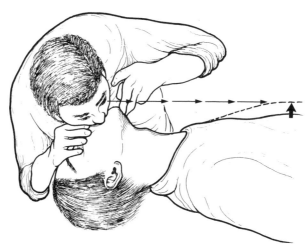

Fig. 5.3   Keeping the chin and neck in the same position as described above, and with the finger and thumb of the right hand pinching the nose, place your lips firmly over the mouth – having taken a large breath – and exhale. Look for the chest rising as you exhale. Next, release your seal and wait for the passive exhalation, again checking that the chest is moving. Repeat the process once exhalation is complete; this usually means about 12–15 breaths per minute.

Oronasal resuscitation

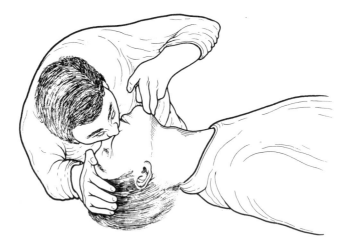

Fig. 5.4   Frequently, it is more desirable to use the nose as the airway, particularly if you cannot get an airtight seal over the mouth or if the mouth contains blood or vomit. Use the left hand to hold the chin forwards and upwards and to keep the mouth shut. If this is not possible, use a pad over the mouth to seal it. Place your mouth over the entire nose and exhale. Then follow the same procedure as for mouth-to-mouth resuscitation.

CIRCULATION
External cardiac massage

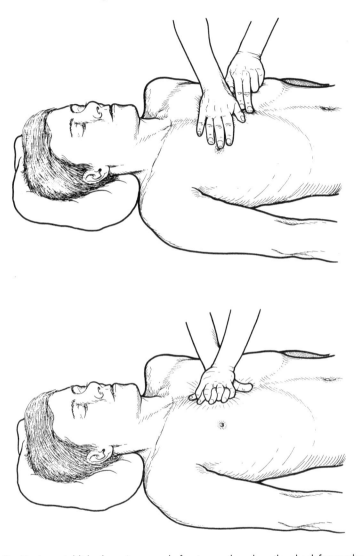

Fig. 5.5   Having established an airway and after two or three breaths, check for a pulse. If it is absent, start external cardiac massage. Place the heel of the right hand over the sternum 3–4 cm above the xiphisternum and place the left hand on top. Keeping the arms straight, compress the sternum by 5 cm and then release; ensure that compression occupies at least half of the cycle. Repeat the cycle 60–80 times per minute. If you are working single-handed, then 15 compressions to two inflations is the method to use.

Advanced resuscitation

Advanced resuscitation follows on from basic CPR and involves recognition of the cardiac dysrhythmia. This section shows three flow diagrams for the three major cardiac abnormalities. Our aim is to describe the restoration of cardiac output, not the treatment of any underlying illness.

Familiarity with the equipment is essential, particularly with relation to the defibrillator and how it is charged and discharged.

(The flow diagrams were produced by the Resuscitation Council, and we are grateful to the Editor of the British Medical Journal for permission to print them.)

Position

The patient is supine. The airway is protected by intubation and administration of 100% oxygen. A large bore central venous cannula is in place, or at least a peripheral line. An electrocardiogram (ECG) monitor is connected to the patient and basic CPR performed.

PLACEMENT OF DEFIBRILLATOR PADDLES

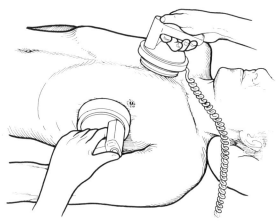

Fig. 5.6   Place one of the paddles below the right clavicle and one just below and lateral to the normal apex beat, i.e. V4 and V5 ECG points; on some defibrillators, the paddles will be marked 'sternum' and 'apex'. The contact between skin and paddle should be firm, with either conducting jelly or adherent conducting pads between them. The machine will indicate when the desired charge is ready. At this point, it is important that all personnel stand back and you should give a command to this effect; then discharge the current by pressing the buttons on the defibrillator paddles.

VENTRICULAR FIBRILLATION

Defibrillate
200 joules (J)
↓
Check pulse
15 compressions
Read ECG
↓
Defibrillate
200 J
↓
Check pulse
15 compressions
Read ECG
↓
Defibrillate
400 J
↓
Check pulse
15 compressions
Read ECG
↓
Give lignocaine 100 mg
↓
Defibrillate
400 J
↓
Check pulse
15 compressions
Read ECG
↓
Give adrenaline 10 ml of
1:10 000
↓
Defibrillate
400 J
↓
Check pulse
15 compressions
Read ECG
↓
Give sodium bicarbonate 50 ml
8.4%
↓
Defibrillate
400 J
↓
Consider further lignocaine,
bretylium or other anti-arrhythmics
Consider changing the position of
the paddles and/or a change of
defibrillator

Fig. 5.7

ASYSTOLE

Atropine 1 mg i.v.
↓
Check pulse
15 compressions
Read ECG
↓
Adrenaline 10 ml of 1:10 000
↓
Check pulse
15 compressions
Read ECG
↓
Sodium bicarbonate 50 ml 8.4%
↓
Check pulse
15 compressions
Read ECG
↓
Isoprenaline 100 μg
↓
Consider intracardiac adrenaline
Consider pacing

Fig. 5.8

ELECTROMECHANICAL DISSOCIATION

Consider causes: Drugs
Cardiac tamponade
Tension pneumothorax
Pulmonary embolus
↓
Adrenaline 10 ml 1:10 000
↓
Check pulse
15 compressions
Read ECG
↓
Isoprenaline 100 μg
↓
Check pulse
15 compressions
Read ECG
↓
Calcium chloride 10 ml 10%

Fig. 5.9   Definition: the presence of QRS complexes in the absence of cardiac output

69

Intracardiac injection

Intracardiac injection is used during resuscitation for the direct administration of drugs.

Equipment
(1) A 16G spinal needle
(2) A 10 ml syringe.

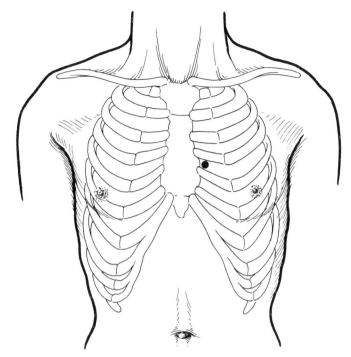

Fig. 5.10A

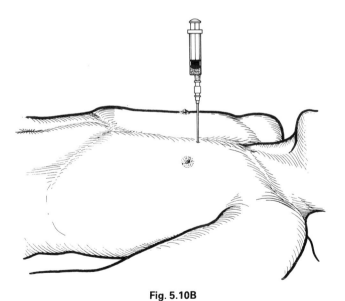

Fig. 5.10B

Fig. 5.10   The site of insertion is at the left sternal edge in the fourth or
fifth intercostal space (A). Insert the needle perpendicular to the skin,
aspirating with advancement (B). When blood is obtained, connect the
syringe containing the drug and inject the drug.

71

Pericardiocentesis

There are two indications for this procedure:
(1) Attempted relief of acute cardiac tamponade in an emergency
(2) To obtain a sample of pericardial fluid for investigation.
Pericardiocentesis is a hazardous technique and should be performed only under supervision in the non-emergency case where echocardiography can be used to confirm the effusion and during the procedure to locate the needle tip.

Position

The patient is supine in the emergency case. For more routine cases, the patient should be sitting in bed at 45°. An earthed ECG machine should be connected to the patient during the procedure.

Equipment

(1) An earthed ECG machine
(2) An 18G Abbocath or equivalent 10 cm central venous cannula
(3) Specimen tubes for cell count, cytology, culture, gram stain and protein.

Management

(1) Constant ECG monitoring
(2) Half-hourly pulse and blood pressure.

Complications

(1) Ventricular puncture
(2) Arrhythmias
(3) Coronary artery injury
(4) Haemopericardium
(5) Cardiac tamponade
(6) Pneumothorax
(7) Infection.

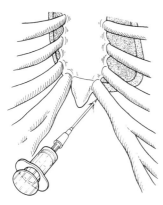

Fig. 5.11 Identify the xiphisternum and clean and drape the surrounding area. Infiltrate local anaesthetic through the skin and beneath the left costal margin. The entry point is in the angle between the xiphisternum and left costal margin. Advance the central venous cannula, connected to a 10 ml syringe, beneath the left costal margin in the angle between it and the xiphisternum.

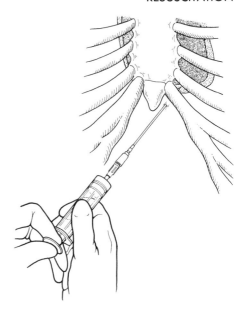

Fig. 5.12 Once the needle is beneath the costal margin, depress the hub of the needle and advance the needle in the direction of the left shoulder. Aspirate with advancement. A 'give' may be felt on going through the pericardial sac. Watch the ECG monitor constantly. The ECG will show arrhythmias which indicate myocardial contact. If this occurs, withdraw the needle by a few millimetres and attempt further aspiration.

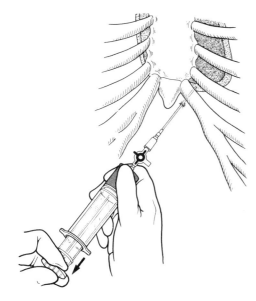

Fig. 5.13 When fluid is obtained, withdraw the needle leaving the cannula in place; connect a three-way tap and aspirate using a 50 ml syringe. Should fluid not be obtained, withdraw the needle and redirect it towards the head or right shoulder.

If bloody fluid is obtained, this suggests cardiac puncture; it can be ascertained by sending the fluid for clotting studies and haematocrit along with venous peripheral blood. If the two are the same, then cardiac puncture is confirmed and you should remove the needle.

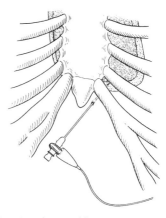

Fig. 5.14 It is also possible to use an 18G spinal needle with an alligator clip connecting the V1 lead to the hub. If the ECG is connected to the needle, then S-T segment elevation indicates ventricular contact and P-R elevation atrial contact; both are indications to withdraw the needle a few millimetres. However in the emergency situation this is usually not possible.

Emergency left thoracotomy

Patients brought into the Accident and Emergency (A & E) department *in extremis* from exsanguination or cardiac tamponade consequent upon penetrating chest injuries, require an emergency thoracotomy. Immediate action with release of acute pericardial tamponade or arrest of bleeding from a cardiac laceration, results in a high incidence of survival in patients who would otherwise succumb.

Catastrophic abdominal haemorrhage can also be controlled by cross-clamping the descending aorta, approached through a left thoracotomy. Suspected cardiac wounds are best approached through a median sternotomy, but the equipment for this is not normally available in the A & E department. This being the case, a left thoracotomy is the next best incision for all wounds except those lateral to the right nipple, which should be approached through a right thoracotomy.

The left thoracotomy will be described here. You may never do it, but *be prepared*. As you start the procedure, call for help from the next senior person.

Position

The patient is in the supine position with a sand-bag placed under the left chest.

Equipment

(1) A size 22 scalpel blade and handle
(2) 3/0 prolene suture on a round-bodied needle
(3) Small Teflon sheets cut into rectangular patches
(4) A large bore Argyll chest drain.

Special points

The sort of patient who requires emergency left thoracotomy often needs no anaesthesia at the outset, but should be intubated and ventilated as the thoracotomy is carried out.

Management

The patient is ventilated after the procedure and transferred to the intensive care unit.

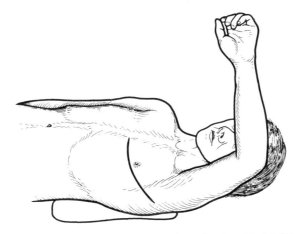

Fig. 5.15   Make an incision along the lower border of the left fifth intercostal space through all the muscles down to the pleura.

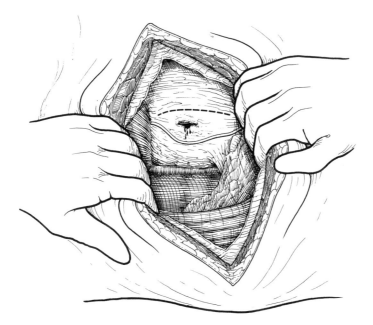

Fig. 5.16   Incise the pleura with the scalpel and get an assistant to retract the rib cage. Push the lung posteriorly with a large pack to expose the left side of the pericardium. Remove blood and clot from the pleural cavity and open the pericardium anterior to the phrenic nerve.

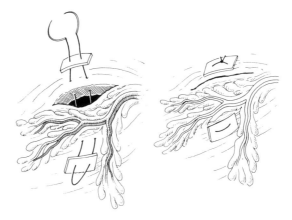

Fig. 5.17   A spurting cardiac wound is controlled by the finger. By this time, skilled help should have arrived, but if not, insert Teflon patches as shown. Major abdominal bleeding can be temporarily controlled by compressing the aorta against the vertebral column just above the diaphragm with the clenched fist until help arrives. An alternative manoeuvre is to cross-clamp the aorta with any soft clamp (even a bowel clamp) as it lies on the posterior thoracic wall.

Heimlich manoeuvre (bear hug)

This manoeuvre is used to relieve acute asphyxiation from impaction of a food or other bolus in the hypopharynx/larynx. This is not a very likely manoeuvre that the house officer will have to deploy while on duty but it is as well to know about it both in the A & E department and while out with your partner at a restaurant.

Clinical features include gasping respiration, clutching at the collar, rapid onset of cyanosis and unconsciousness, and, occasionally, a convulsion.

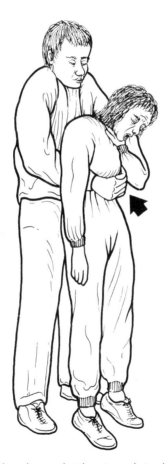

Fig. 5.18   Quickly make sure that there is no obviously impacted denture or piece of food that you can remove by hooking it out with your fingers. Get behind the patient whether he is upright or on the floor. Grasp your arms firmly around his or her lower ribs and across the epigastrium. Then just after the next gasp tighten your grip to give a fierce thrust to the upper abdomen. If nothing happens repeat this every ten seconds for half a minute.

Chapter 6

Respiratory system

Endotracheal intubation

Endotracheal intubation is necessary during general anaesthesia when the patient requires to be 'paralysed', as for thoracic and abdominal operations. It is also used to protect and maintain the airway when access is compromised, as in operations around the head, or indeed, for any lengthy procedure. During resuscitation, endotracheal intubation – in addition to providing a means of direct ventilation – also safeguards the airway from aspiration of stomach contents.

Position

The patient is supine with extension of the atlanto-occipital joint and spine of the cervical flexion. This position can best be described as 'sniffing the morning air'.

Equipment

(1) An endotracheal tube (which should be cut at the 24 cm mark for adults)
(2) A laryngoscope.

Complications

(1) Malposition with intubation of the oesophagus
(2) Compression or stretching of the recurrent laryngeal nerve in difficult procedures (this is usually followed by complete recovery within a few days)
(3) Trauma to the lips, gums, teeth and oropharynx.

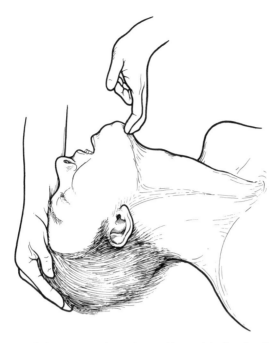

Fig. 6.1   With the patient in the supine position and the head resting on a pillow, place the left hand on the top of the head and push the head backwards and downwards towards the shoulders. This brings the chin up and allows the mouth to drop open.

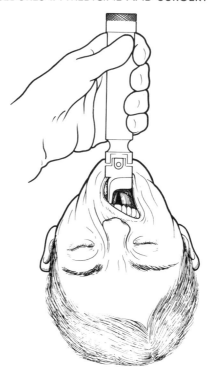

Fig. 6.2   The laryngoscope is a left-handed instrument. Hold it in the palm of the hand, as shown, and insert into the right-hand side of the mouth to allow the blade to move the tongue to the left and thus out of the way. After passing it through into the pharynx, you will see the epiglottis covering part of the vocal cords and obscuring the aperture into the larynx. The larynx lies anterior to the oesophagus with the pyriform fossae on each side.

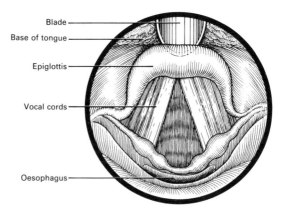

Fig. 6.3   Place the tip of the laryngoscope anterior to the epiglottis at the base of the tongue and lift it upwards and distally with the handle pointing approximately 45° away from you. This raises the epiglottis and reveals the vocal cords. The laryngoscope is not inserted over the epiglottis because the lower part receives some fibres from the vagus nerve and excessive stimulation may lead to cardiac arrhythmias. Take care during this part of the procedure to avoid damaging the incisors.

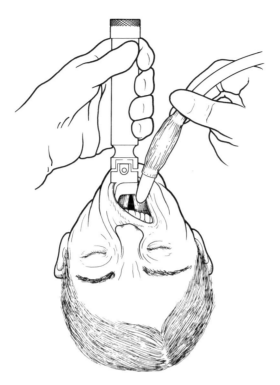

Fig. 6.4   Enter the lubricated endotracheal tube into the pharynx from the right side, so that vision of the vocal cords is not obscured, and insert it through the vocal aperture and into the larynx.

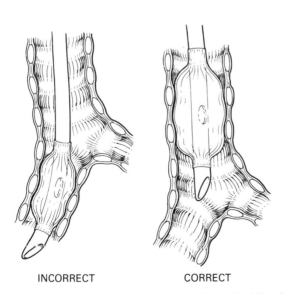

INCORRECT   CORRECT

Fig. 6.5   Push the tube distally into the trachea, where it should lie above the carina as shown. If the tube is inserted too far, it will prevent ventilation of one lung and you *must* check for this by auscultation of the chest after insertion. Inflate the balloon and secure the tube by placing it in the corner of the mouth and tying a soft tape around the neck.

Urgent tracheostomy

Tracheostomy done hurriedly in circumstances of near complete or complete upper airway obstruction rarely saves life. Intubation (see p. 80 should be carried out wherever possible, and if this fails, a laryngotomy performed (see p. 86).

Subsequent to successful intubation, a decision rarely may be taken to establish a tracheostomy immediately. This procedure should not be performed by unsupervised junior staff.

Position

The patient is supine with a sand-bag under the shoulders (a litre bag of intravenous fluid will suffice) and the neck extended.

Equipment

(1) A scalpel and a size 10 blade
(2) Toothed forceps
(3) A tracheostomy tube and syringe to inflate the balloon.

Complications

(1) Bleeding, sometimes from the thyroid isthmus
(2) Inadequate insertion of the tracheostomy tube.

Management

When in position, the tracheostomy tube is secured by tying a tape around the neck. A gauze pad should be placed between the external part of the tube and the skin, and this should be changed daily. If the tracheostomy is required for more than 10 days, it can be replaced by a 'silver tube' once the patient is conscious and breathing spontaneously. The silver tubes are changed and cleaned daily. Before removing the silver tube, the trachea is aspirated to remove any mucus and the suction tube must remain in hand. The silver tube is lifted out and its replacement inserted. Providing that this is not performed too early (i.e. less than one week after tracheostomy formation), a track will have been formed along which the silver tube can pass.

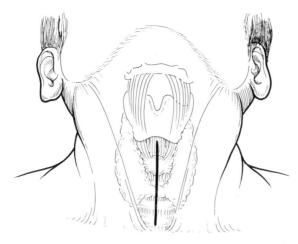

Fig. 6.6 With the patient's neck extended, make an incision from the lower border of the thyroid cartilage to the suprasternal notch. A vertical incision is recommended; all tracheostomy incisions heal to a small rounded scar so that it is not usually possible to tell vertical from transverse, and there is less bleeding from a vertical incision.

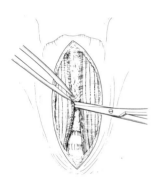

Fig. 6.7 Continue the incision through the deep investing fascia of the neck down to the strap muscles, which should be split in the midline to expose the loose areolar tissue around the thyroid isthmus and the front of the trachea.

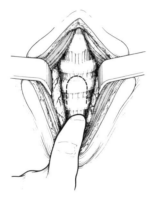

Fig. 6.8 By means of blunt dissection using a finger, bare the trachea by sweeping all structures either upwards or downwards. This manoeuvre will move the thyroid isthmus out of the area; it rarely, if ever, requires formal dissection and division. Identify the second or third tracheal ring by counting down from the cricoid cartilage, and make an inverted U incision.

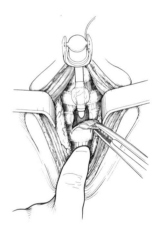

Fig. 6.9 Pick up the tip of this flap with toothed forceps and insert the tracheostomy tube. Once the balloon has been inflated and adequate ventilation confirmed, ligate any bleeding points and suture the tip of the inverted U flap to the subcutaneous tissue. This maintains access to the trachea if the tube becomes dislodged. Use an absorbable suture, to close the deep fascia, and approximate the skin with 3/0 interrupted nylon.

Emergency laryngotomy

This is performed as an emergency procedure in order to maintain the airway. It may be usefully preceded by thrusting one or more 16G needles through the cricothyroid membrane, as even this narrow passage will allow some gas exchange. Formal equipment may not be available, in which case, a penknife and a hollow tube (such as a ball-point pen) will suffice. All the steps described below must be carried out with speed. Should you use a makeshift tube, it must be held in place until control can be gained by more secure means.

Position

The patient is supine with the neck extended.

Equipment

(1) A scalpel with a size 10 blade
(2) A paediatric size tracheal tube.

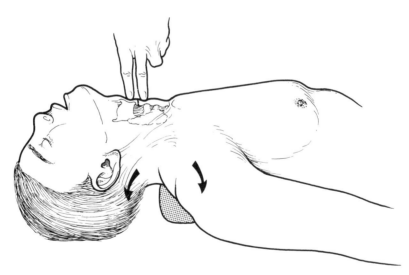

Fig. 6.10   Without anaesthetic or skin preparation, palpate the gap between the thyroid and cricoid cartilages. Place a finger on either side of the gap.

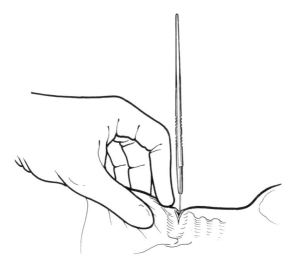

Fig. 6.11   Grasping the thyroid cartilage with the thumb and middle finger, use the index finger to palpate the gap. Make a horizontal skin incision over the gap at the tip of the index finger, and then with a stabbing movement push the scalpel blade through into the larynx.

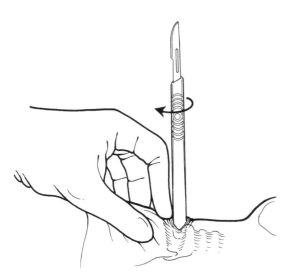

Fig. 6.12   Reverse the scalpel and push the handle into the larynx. Rotate the handle through 90° to enlarge the opening.

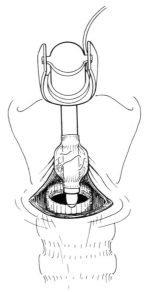

Fig. 6.13   Immediately insert the tube through the opening and attach it to an Ambu bag.

The Sellick manoeuvre (cricoid pressure)

Emergency induction and intubation in a patient who may have a full stomach carries with it the risk of regurgitation of stomach contents with aspiration into the chest. For this reason, every emergency induction and intubation must be accompanied by pressure on the cricoid cartilage, which occludes the upper end of the oesophagus thus preventing regurgitation.

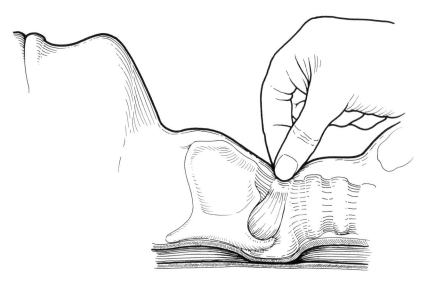

Fig. 6.14   Before the patient has been anaesthetized, get *the assistant* to locate the cricoid cartilage by gentle palpation and to 'pinch' it between the forefinger and thumb. The moment the patient is anaesthetized, push the cricoid cartilage firmly backwards. This manoeuvre occludes the oesophagus as demonstrated.

Chapter 7

Pleural cavity

Thoracentesis

Fluid is aspirated from the pleural cavity for both diagnostic and therapeutic purposes.

Position

The patient should be sitting upright, with the arms forward over a rest (as shown in Fig. 7.1).

The site for aspiration is usually posterior between the medial border of the scapula and the spine, the level depending on the level of fluid as determined by clinical and radiological examination.

Equipment

(1) A large bore intravenous cannula (14G or 16G) with a needle and syringe
(2) A three-way tap.

Complications

(1) Pneumothorax
(2) Damage to lung parenchyma
(3) Damage to intraperitoneal structures if the needle is inserted too low (the liver on the right and the spleen on the left are particularly vulnerable).

Management

Once the procedure is finished, the cannula is removed and a dry dressing placed over the puncture site. A flexible collodion solution assists in making the seal air-tight.

Fluid may be sent for biochemical (protein and glucose), bacteriological and cytological analyses.

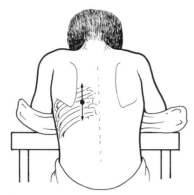

Fig. 7.1   Position the patient in the sitting position with the arms placed over a rest, as illustrated. The approach is from the posterior aspect, approximately halfway between the medial border of the scapula and the spine.

   After skin preparation, infiltrate local anaesthesia into the lower part of the intercostal space chosen, down to and through the pleura until fluid can be withdrawn.

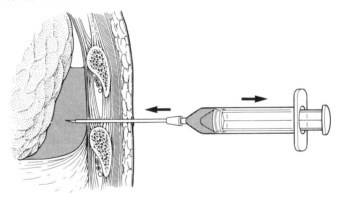

Fig. 7.2   Insert the intravenous cannula and needle with syringe just above the rib of the chosen intercostal space until fluid is withdrawn. Advance the cannula over the needle and withdraw the latter. The syringe has to be removed temporarily to allow the needle to be withdrawn and care must be taken not to allow air into the pleural cavity. This should not occur if the cannula remains within the pleural effusion fluid.

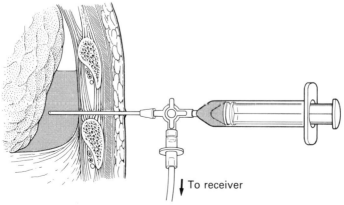

To receiver

91

Fig. 7.3   If large amounts of fluid are to be aspirated, insert a three-way tap with a length of tubing (part of an intravenous administration set is useful for this), to allow drainage of fluid directly into a receiver.

Pleural biopsy

Pleural biopsy can be performed at the same time as thoracentesis, and obtaining pleural tissue in the presence of a pleural effusion is relatively straightforward. The same is not true for pleural biopsy without an effusion, and this procedure should not be performed by junior staff without supervision.

Position
The patient is positioned as for thoracentesis (see Fig. 7.1).

Equipment
Abrams' pleural biopsy needle.

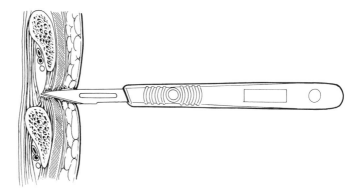

Fig. 7.4   After skin preparation and local anaesthetic infiltration over the chosen intercostal space, make a small incision in the skin using a size 11 scalpel blade and extend it through the intercostal muscles for approximately 1 cm.

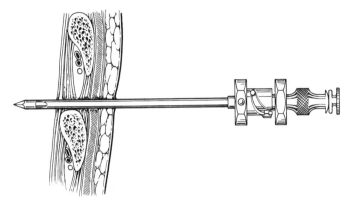

Fig. 7.5   Insert the Abrams' needle until the characteristic 'give' is felt as the pleural cavity is entered.

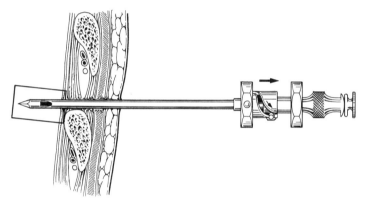

Fig. 7.6   Withdraw the inner trocar slightly by turning it anti-clockwise to expose the biopsy port.

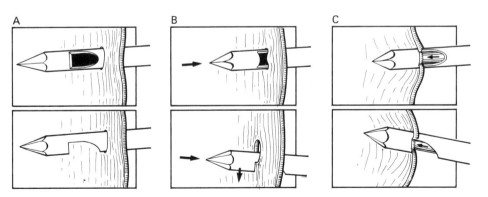

Fig. 7.7   Expose the biopsy mechanism (A). Turn the instrument so that the biopsy mechanism faces downwards (B). This prevents possible damage to the intercostal vessels and nerves which are lying superiorly. Withdraw the needle slowly until the parietal pleura is felt to 'catch'. Close the trocar by turning it clockwise and remove the whole needle in one movement (C). This procedure should be repeated two or three times in order to obtain adequate samples for histological analysis.

93

Insertion of a chest drain

Traumatic or spontaneous injuries to the chest resulting in either a pneumothorax or haemothorax, require drainage. In both elective and emergency situations, this is best performed under direct vision by the 'open' method described here.

Position

The patient may be either supine (usually in the emergency situation and in the unconscious patient) or sitting upright, with the arms forward over a rest (as shown in (Fig. 7.8).
    The site of insertion may be:

(1) The second intercostal space, mid-clavicular line
(2) The fifth intercostal space, mid-axillary line.

The second intercostal space is usually reserved for drainage of a pneumothorax, whereas the mid-axillary approach can be used for draining both blood and air, depending on the angle with which the drainage tube is inserted (see Fig. 7.10). The latter approach will be described here but the principles are the same for the anterior approach.

Equipment

(1) A scalpel and a size 10 blade
(2) An Argyle (Definition of Sherwood Medical, Tullamore, Ireland) chest drain (the sizes vary from 18 ch to 32 ch). When the drain is inserted for trauma the largest size possible (usually 32) should be inserted.
(3) An underwater drainage system
(4) 100 ml of water for the drainage bottle.

Complications

(1) Damage to underlying lung parenchyma by an unguarded thrust of the trocar (this complication is highly unlikely if the pleura is approached under direct vision as described here).
(2) Damage to the intercostal vessels and nerve
(3) Damage to the long thoracic nerve (of Bell) which supplies the serratus anterior muscle. This nerve runs down the medial wall of the axilla posterior to the mid-axillary line.

Management

(1) A post-insertion chest x-ray is mandatory.
(2) The end of the tubing in the underwater system must always be under water to prevent air from entering the pleural cavity, and the water within the tube must swing with respiration – indicating patency.
(3) The underwater system should be kept below the patient, usually on the floor. When the patient is moved about the hospital, and providing that there is not an air leak, the tube is clamped.

(4) Suction may be applied to the exit tubing of the underwater system if required to aid the re-expansion of a resistant pneumothorax, or to drain pleural fluid collections such as occur following thoracic surgery.

Removal

The drain is removed after deep inspiration, which reduces the potential space within the pleural cavity. The purse string, positioned at the time of insertion, is drawn tight and tied.

Removal of the chest drain should always be followed by an erect chest x-ray to confirm that a pneumothorax does not remain.

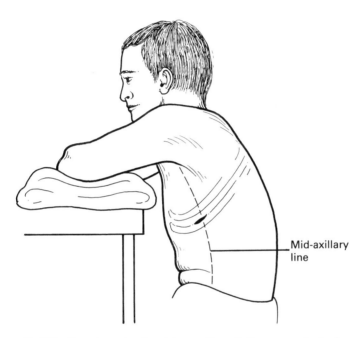

Mid-axillary line

Fig. 7.8   Place the patient in a sitting position with the arms semi-raised over a rest – this can be a table with one or two pillows on top. Infiltrate local anaesthetic over the planned line of incision. Here, the incision is over the lower part of the fifth intercostal space in the mid-axillary line for approximately 3 cm.

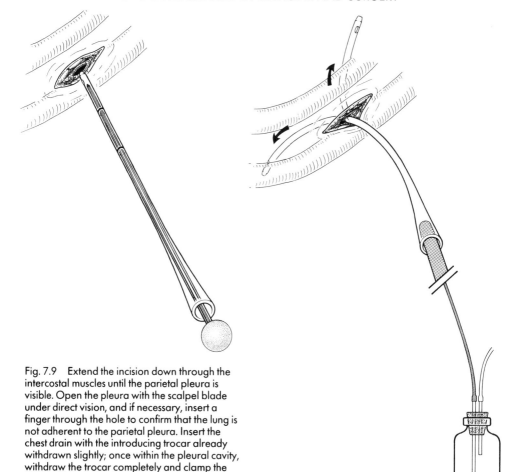

Fig. 7.9 Extend the incision down through the intercostal muscles until the parietal pleura is visible. Open the pleura with the scalpel blade under direct vision, and if necessary, insert a finger through the hole to confirm that the lung is not adherent to the parietal pleura. Insert the chest drain with the introducing trocar already withdrawn slightly; once within the pleural cavity, withdraw the trocar completely and clamp the drain. 'Blind' insertion of a chest drain should not be done.

Fig. 7.10 Once the drain is in position, directed upwards for a pneumothorax or downwards for a haemothorax, connect it to the underwater system.

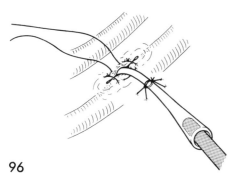

Fig. 7.11 Close the wound with a single layer of interrupted 2/0 nylon sutures. Fix the drain securely by suturing it to the skin on each side with No 1 nylon on a cutting needle. This allows equal pull to be exerted on the drain, which results in greater security and less discomfort in the postoperative period. Finally, place a purse string suture (3/0) around the drain but leave it untied. This allows closure of the wound when the drain is removed. An absorbent dressing is placed over the wound.

Chapter 8

Peritoneal cavity

Abdominal paracentesis

Abdominal paracentesis is a diagnostic and therapeutic procedure in the management of patients with ascites. It is a relatively straightforward procedure which can be performed on the ward under sterile conditions.

Position

The patient is supine with a slightly lateral inclination in order to collect the most amount of ascitic fluid in an area where insertion of the catheter is least likely to cause damage (right or left iliac fossa).

Equipment

(1) A large bore intravenous cannula (size 14–16G)
(2) A 20 ml syringe
(3) A three-way tap
(4) Rubber tubing (or an intravenous administration set)
(5) A receiver.

Complications

(1) Damage to underlying viscera is unlikely using a needle of this size.
(2) If a large amount of liquid is removed, it may be replaced rapidly in the peritoneal cavity from the patient's extracellular space. This complication can be avoided by sequential aspirations on a daily basis, or better by concomitant intravenous fluid replacement.

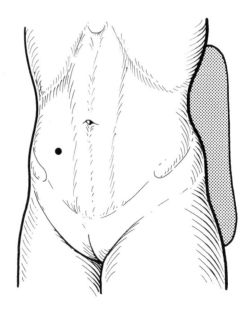

Fig. 8.1   Clean the area of insertion (through a point lying two thirds of the way along a line between the umbilicus and the anterior superior iliac spine), and infiltrate local anaesthesia down to the peritoneum.

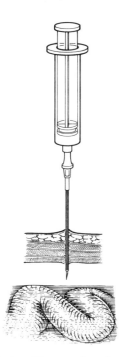

Fig. 8.2 Insert the cannula and needle with the attached syringe into the peritoneal cavity at right angles to the skin.

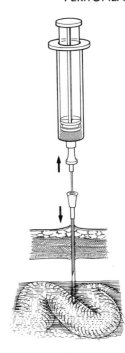

Fig. 8.3 When ascitic fluid is withdrawn, gently advance the cannula over the needle, which is then removed.

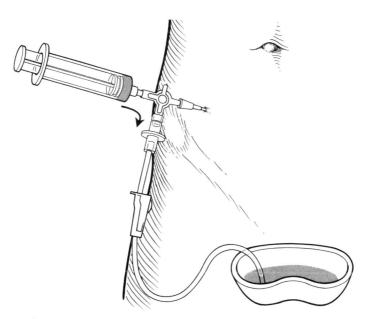

Fig. 8.4 If large quantities of fluid are to be withdrawn, attach the three-way tap with the rubber tubing. This allows repeated aspiration and drainage to be performed. Recurrent aspirations are better managed by the insertion of a peritoneal dialysis catheter, as described under 'peritoneal lavage' (see p. 100).

Peritoneal lavage

Peritoneal lavage has now superseded abdominal paracentesis and the 'four quadrant tap' as the investigation of choice in blunt abdominal trauma. It has a very high sensitivity for the detection of intraperitoneal bleeding and should be performed in the A & E department under sterile conditions. The patient must always be catheterized before the procedure.

Position

The patient should be supine with the head down.

Equipment

(1) A catheter (the same as for peritoneal dialysis) with a trocar
(2) 1 litre of normal saline with a giving set
(3) A scalpel with a size 10 blade
(4) A small self-retaining retractor (West or Traver's).

Complications

(1) Bleeding from the wound
(2) Damage to underlying structures, namely bowel, bladder, mesentery and major vessels. This should be kept to a minimum if the peritoneum is opened under direct vision.

Special points

(1) The fluid is tested for red blood cell (RBC) and white blood cell (WBC) concentration, amylase content and the presence of bile-stained fluid or bacteria (urgent gram stain).
(2) The usual indications for laparotomy following blunt abdominal trauma are[1]:
    (i)   RBC concentration >100 000/mm^3
    (ii)   WBC concentration >500/mm^3
    (iii) Amylase concentration >200 units/100 mm^3.
(3) If the results fall into the indeterminate range (see below), the lavage should be repeated after 1–2 hours.
    (i)   RBC concentration 50–100 000/mm^3
    (ii)   WBC concentration 100–500/mm^3
    (iii) Amylase concentration 75–200 units/100 mm^3.

[1] Alyono D., Perry J. F. (1981). 'Value of quantitative cell count and amylase activity of peritoneal lavage fluid'. J. Trauma, 21, 345.

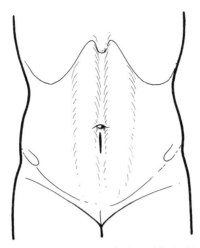

Fig. 8.5 Infiltrate local anaesthesia in the line of the incision down to the peritoneum. Make a vertical incision approximately 5 cm long below the umbilicus in the midline.

Fig. 8.6 Using a self-retaining retractor, extend this incision down through the linea alba. After picking up the peritoneum between two artery forceps, make a small incision through it and insert the catheter under direct vision, with the trocar slightly withdrawn.

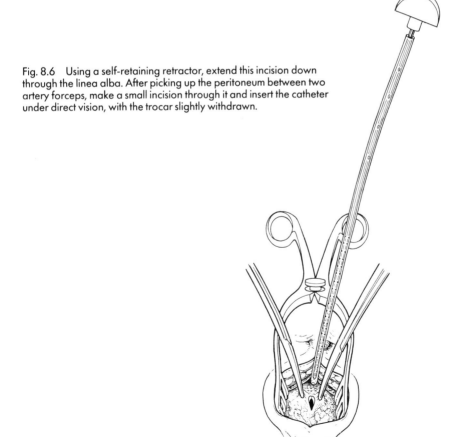

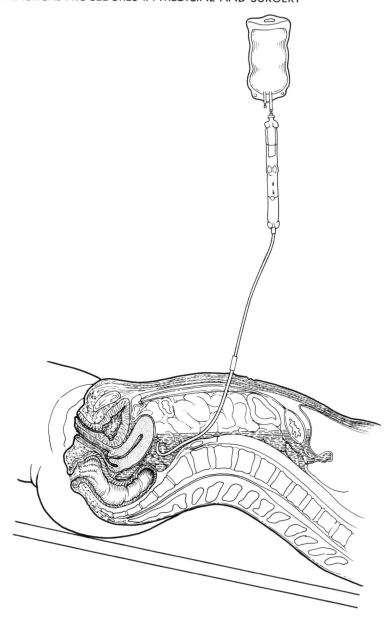

Fig. 8.7 Withdraw the trocar completely and gently push the catheter down into the pelvis. Secure the catheter to the skin with a suture connected to the intravenous giving set, and immediately infuse 1 litre of normal saline into the peritoneal cavity.

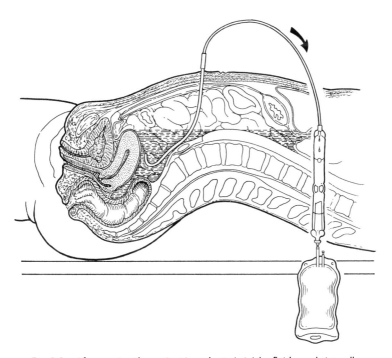

Fig. 8.8   After moving the patient in order to 'mix' the fluid evenly into all four quadrants of the peritoneal cavity, place the empty bag on the floor to allow the peritoneal fluid to return into it. After completing the procedure, suture the wound and either leave the catheter in situ or remove it, depending on whether a repeat lavage is to be performed later.

Gastro-intestinal system

Insertion of a nasogastric tube

This is a frequently requested procedure that is not usually carried out by the junior doctor. However, he is often summoned when difficulty arises. It is sensible, therefore, to be proficient and to have had practice in easier circumstances.

Explain to the patient what you are going to do and what you expect from them as this is an unpleasant procedure.

Position

The patient should be sitting comfortably in bed. Ask the patient if either of his nostrils is blocked or if there is any difficulty in nasal breathing.

Equipment

(1) A nasogastric tube (from the fridge)
(2) A glass of water
(3) Lubricating jelly
(4) A bladder syringe or 50 ml syringe, depending on the size of the tube and its connections
(5) Adhesive tape.

Management

The position of the tube should be checked by x-ray if doubt exists. The position should be checked daily, paying attention to the markers.

Complications

(1) Tracheal intubation
(2) Aspiration
(3) Oesophagitis, erosion and stricture
(4) Nasal erosion
(5) Nose bleed.

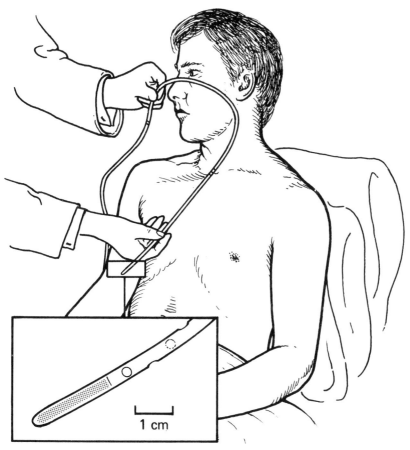

Fig. 9.1   Holding the tube against the patient, estimate the length of tube
necessary to enter the stomach; this is approximately 50 cm.

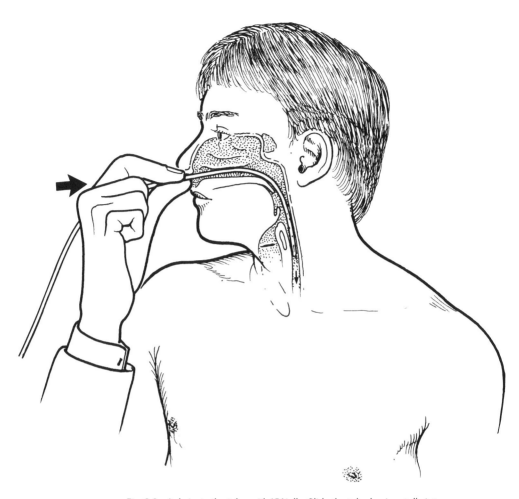

Fig. 9.2   Lubricate the tube with KY jelly. Slide the tube horizontally into the nostril and ask the patient when he feels it at the back of the 'throat'. Resist the temptation to push the tube *upwards* — the floor of the nasal cavity is horizontal and the tube should follow this. Advance the tube down the oesophagus. With each advancement, ask the patient to swallow; this is helped by allowing the patient to take a sip of water as swallowing is difficult with a dry mouth. If the patient gags excessively, encourage him to take deep breaths through the mouth while advancing the tube.

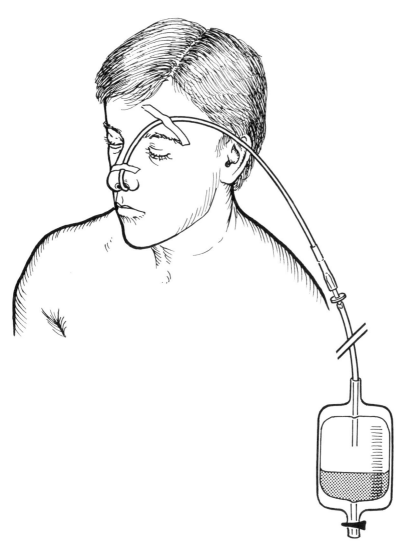

Fig. 9.3   When the desired length has been inserted, test that it is in the stomach by blowing 50 ml of air down the tube with the syringe while listening with a stethoscope under the left costal margin. A definite bubbling noise is heard if the tube is correctly placed. Once the tube is in the right place, tape it into position at the nose and on the forehead. Make a mark on the tube so that movement can be detected easily. Aspirate the stomach and connect the tube to a drainage bag if free drainage is required; otherwise, it should be spigotted.

Gastric lavage

Gastric lavage is used in the A & E department to empty a patient's stomach following an overdose of oral drugs. It is also used on the surgical wards to empty the stomach of patients due to undergo surgery for pyloric stenosis. The following description is for lavage following an overdose. This procedure requires two people. If the patient is unconscious or has a depressed 'gag' reflex, endotracheal intubation (see p. 80) should be carried out before lavage.

Position

The patient lies on his left or right side with a 20° head down tilt, although when gastric lavage is performed before surgery the patient can be sitting at 45°. The patient and staff should have waterproof protection!

Equipment

(1) A 34Ch gastric tube
(2) A 140 ml syringe
(3) A bucket half filled with tap water
(4) Plastic sheets
(5) Suction equipment
(6) A 250 ml jug.

Complications

(1) Intratracheal intubation
(2) Aspiration pneumonitis.

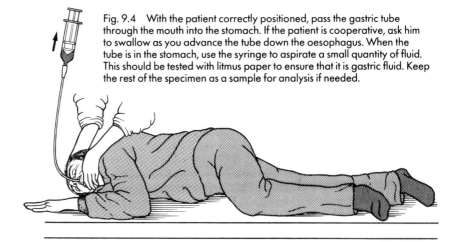

Fig. 9.4   With the patient correctly positioned, pass the gastric tube through the mouth into the stomach. If the patient is cooperative, ask him to swallow as you advance the tube down the oesophagus. When the tube is in the stomach, use the syringe to aspirate a small quantity of fluid. This should be tested with litmus paper to ensure that it is gastric fluid. Keep the rest of the specimen as a sample for analysis if needed.

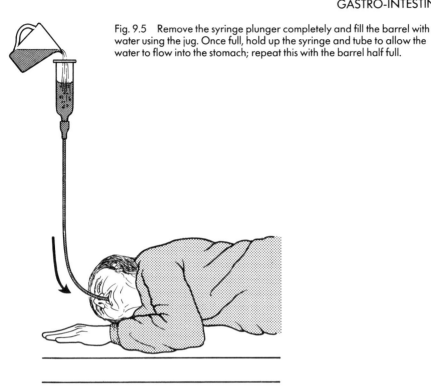

Fig. 9.5   Remove the syringe plunger completely and fill the barrel with water using the jug. Once full, hold up the syringe and tube to allow the water to flow into the stomach; repeat this with the barrel half full.

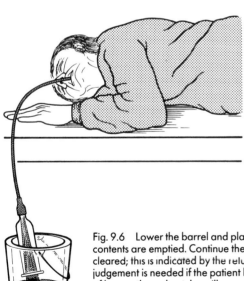

Fig. 9.6   Lower the barrel and place it in the bucket so that the gastric contents are emptied. Continue the lavage until the stomach has been cleared; this is indicated by the return of the clear fluid, although some judgement is needed if the patient has recently eaten because no amount of lavage through a tube will remove all chewed, undigested food. The plunger should be reconnected only to unblock the tube. The tube may be used at the end of the procedure to instil medication or charcoal.

Insertion of a Minnesota (modified Blakemore-Sengstaken) tube

Oesophageal tamponade still has a place in the management of bleeding varices. The procedure is not without risk and should be carried out by junior hospital doctors only in the presence of senior staff. It is technically difficult and potentially dangerous, and best performed by an endoscopist, who will be experienced in intubating the oesophagus. Patients require sedation with diazepam and the clinician must be prepared to perform the procedure under general anaesthesia in extreme cases although this is not common.

Position

The patient is placed in the left lateral position as for upper gastro-intestinal endoscopy.

Equipment

(1) A Minnesota tube. This has four channels, one each for the oesophageal and stomach balloons and another two for gastric and oesophageal aspiration. The Blakemore-Sengstaken tube differs in that it does not have a channel for oesophageal aspiration, and it has probably been superseded by the Minnesota tube.
(2) A low pressure suction pump.

Management

A thoraco-abdominal x-ray should always be taken after the procedure to confirm the correct positioning of the balloons. The patient is managed in a 45° head up tilt, to decrease the risk of aspiration.

The oesophageal aspiration channel should be connected to the suction pump, which is maintained on continual low pressure suction. The gastric aspiration channel is drained by continuous dependent drainage.

When the tube is secured to the cheek, it is important that a soft dressing (foam rubber is suitable) is inserted between the tube and the skin of the cheek to prevent ulceration at the angle of the mouth.

Complications

(1) Malposition
(2) Aspiration of blood.

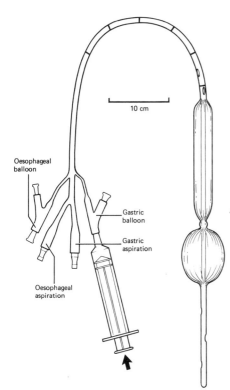

Oesophageal
balloon

Gastric
balloon

Gastric
aspiration

Oesophageal
aspiration

10 cm

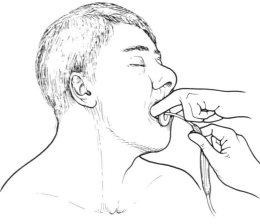

Fig. 9.8   Place the patient in the left lateral position, as for upper gastro-intestinal endoscopy; raise the head to 45° and insert a mouth guard. After spraying the pharynx with local anaesthetic, lubricate the tube with water-soluble jelly and insert it into the pharynx with the right hand, positioning the index and middle finger of the left hand on each side of the mouth guard to direct the tube into the oesophagus.

Fig. 9.7   Ensure that the Minnesota tube is kept in a refrigerator to maintain rigidity — which simplifies insertion. You can use guide wires to strengthen the tube but these are often difficult to remove and are not recommended. Before insertion, inflate the gastric (250–300 ml) and oesophageal (120 ml) balloons with air to confirm patency, as demonstrated.

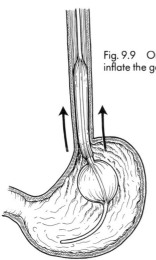

Fig. 9.9   Once the tube is in the stomach, inflate the gastric balloon fully.

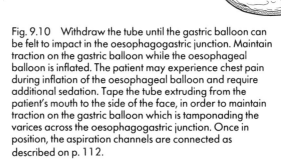

Fig. 9.10   Withdraw the tube until the gastric balloon can be felt to impact in the oesophagogastric junction. Maintain traction on the gastric balloon while the oesophageal balloon is inflated. The patient may experience chest pain during inflation of the oesophageal balloon and require additional sedation. Tape the tube extruding from the patient's mouth to the side of the face, in order to maintain traction on the gastric balloon which is tamponading the varices across the oesophagogastric junction. Once in position, the aspiration channels are connected as described on p. 112.

113

Rectal examination

Examination of the rectum is a three-stage event: digital examination, proctoscopy and sigmoidoscopy.

Position

This is the same for digital examination, proctoscopy and sigmoidoscopy. The patient lies in the left lateral position with the hips and knees flexed. The left hand of the operator raises the patient's right buttock to expose the perianal region which should be carefully examined before any internal examination. The operator should wear gloves at all times.

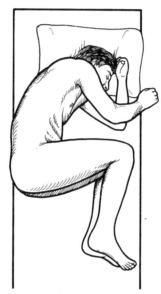

Fig. 9.11   Position the patient in the left lateral position, as shown.

DIGITAL EXAMINATION

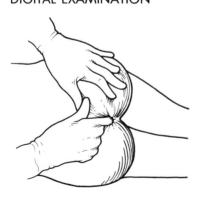

Fig. 9.12   Lubricate your right index finger and insert it into the anal canal by running it anterior to posterior, as illustrated. Systematically palpate all four quadrants, particularly noting the following:

(1)   The perianal condition
(2)   The tone of the anal sphincter
(3)   The presence of acute pain on insertion of the digit, usually indicating the presence of an anal fissure. If this occurs – desist.
(4)   The faeces – presence and consistency
(5)   The rectal mucosa – polyps and tumours
(6)   The prostate gland in men, and the cervix in women
(7)   Extrarectal masses anterior and lateral to the rectum
(8)   Areas of tenderness on palpation
(9)   The colour of the faeces on removing the finger, noting the presence of blood or mucus.

PROCTOSCOPY

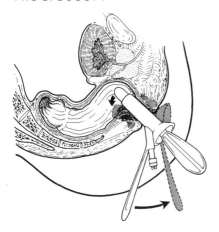

Fig. 9.13   Lubricate the proctoscope and insert it into the anal canal angled anteriorly towards the patient's umbilicus. This is because the anal canal runs from anterior to posterior, as shown. Once inserted, remove the obturator, attach the light source and examine the lower part of the rectum and anal canal. Then gently withdraw the instrument, noting as the anorectal verge is traversed if there is any mucosal redundancy, prolapse or bleeding.

SIGMOIDOSCOPY

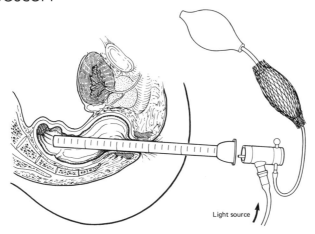

Light source

Fig. 9.14   Insert the instrument through the anal canal in the same way as for proctoscopy. Once the anal canal has been negotiated, remove the obturator, slant the sigmoidoscope back towards the longitudinal axis of the distal rectum and insufflate air to distend the rectal wall. Faeces are often encountered. If they are solid, the sigmoidoscope can sometimes be manipulated past them. If the lumen is not obscured, it may be possible to advance the instrument. Traversing the rectosigmoid junction may be difficult; insufflating air distends the proximal rectum and allows proximal advance. An acute angulation forward of the tip of the instrument is needed to clear the sacral promontory. This may prove impossible if there is colonic impaction.

RECTAL BIOPSY

Fig. 9.15   If a rectal biopsy is required, insert the biopsy forceps through the sigmoidoscope and grasp the rectal mucosa, pulling gently to ascertain that only mucosa is caught. Close the forceps tightly and remove the piece of mucosa. Place the biopsy specimen onto a square of blotting paper and then into a container with formal saline. The blotting paper prevents distortion of the small piece of mucosa, thus aiding subsequent histological examination.

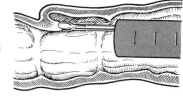

Urogenital system

Urinary catheterization

Insertion of a urinary catheter allows free drainage of urine in cases of urinary retention. It also permits regular monitoring of a patient's urinary output, which provides essential information on the circulating volume and renal function after an operation, on the intensive care unit and during resuscitation following major circulatory collapse. Catheterization is also indicated after deep pelvic dissections where neurological mechanisms of micturition may have been disturbed.

Equipment

(1) Sterile towels (two) and swabs
(2) A urinary catheter (size 16–18G for men and 14G for women)
(3) Chlorhexidine solution and a container.
(4) Lignocaine jelly with a plastic introducer (this usually comes in a sealed packet with an applicator)
(5) A receiver
(6) A syringe with enough water to fill the catheter balloon (the volume varies between 5 ml and 30 ml and is usually marked on the catheter)
(7) A drainage bag.

Position

Men should be supine.
Women should be supine with the ankles placed together, the knees flexed and the hips abducted.

Special points

It is usually said that catheterization of a male with benign prostatic hypertrophy is difficult and prone to failure. In fact, this is not so provided that, as in all circumstances where a catheter is to be passed, the patient is adequately prepared – by reassurance, sedation and lubrication. Except in prostatic cancer, the prostatic urethra is soft, and indeed oedema may be the precipitating event in acute or acute on chronic retention. In circumstances where prostatic hypertrophy is not present, the only difficulty is likely to be from sphincter spasm, which can be prevented by gentle techniques, or from urethral strictures.

Complications

Gentle technique prevents nearly all of these. Urethral stricture may lead to failure with or without bleeding. Suprapubic tap (see p. 124) should then be undertaken, rather than repeated attempts with ever more rigid instruments which may well create a 'false passage' – i.e. a blind, extramucosal tract which is the starting point of para-urethral sepsis.

In women, the only significant cause of failure is that the urethral orifice cannot be identified because of obesity or scarring. A good light and an assistant are essential for success.

PROCEDURE IN MEN

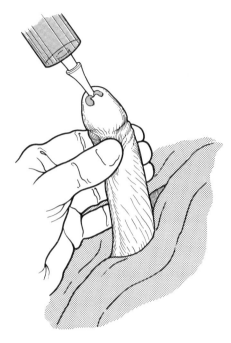

Fig. 10.1   Swab the penis and surrounding skin with chlorhexidine solution and drape the area leaving the penis exposed. Retract the foreskin, if it is present, and clean the glans. Hold the penis at right angles to the body, gently empty a tube of lignocaine jelly into the urethra and massage proximally.

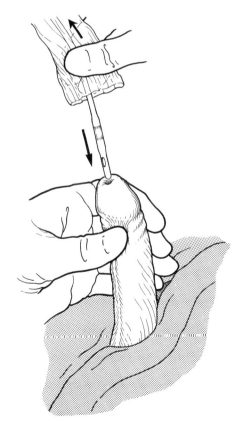

Fig. 10.2   Gently squeeze the urethra to prevent the jelly from flowing out. Insert the catheter tip into the urethral orifice, maintaining the shield of the outer plastic covering. Gradually remove the cover while inserting the catheter gently but steadily further into the urethra. This ensures that the catheter remains sterile throughout the procedure.

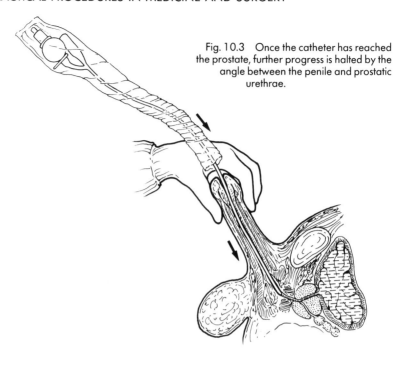

Fig. 10.3   Once the catheter has reached the prostate, further progress is halted by the angle between the penile and prostatic urethrae.

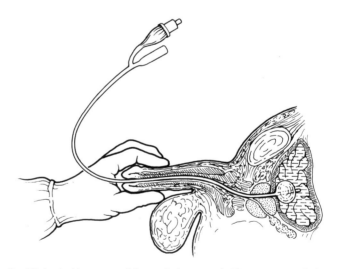

Fig. 10.4   At this stage, pull the penis downwards. This manoeuvre helps to reduce the angle, allowing the catheter to be pushed past the prostate and into the bladder. Now fill the balloon with the required volume of water and withdraw it gently until you feel it rest at the internal urethral orifice; attach the drainage bag to the catheter. The catheter should be inserted to the hilt in order to ensure that the balloon is within the bladder before it is filled.

PROCEDURE IN WOMEN

This technique differs only slightly from that in men. The urethra is only about 1–2 cm long in women and lignocaine jelly is not required, although the catheter tip should be wiped with lubricant before insertion.

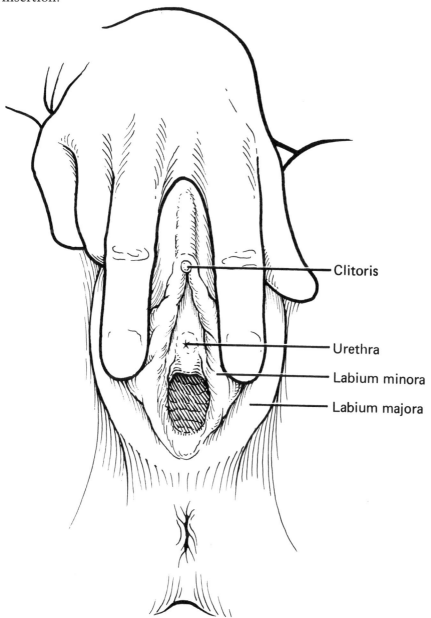

Fig. 10.5   Clean the labia majora and surrounding skin with chlorhexidine solution and drape the surrounding area to expose the labia. Part the labia majora and minora to reveal the urethral orifice, which lies behind the clitoris in the anterior wall of the vagina. After cleaning the urethral orifice, insert the catheter and press it home until urine flows.

REMOVAL OF A URETHRAL CATHETER

In order to remove the catheter, the water in the balloon must first be withdrawn. Occasionally, this is not possible because the narrow channel through which the water was inserted has become blocked. The first manoeuvre is to insert a small volume of water (1–2 ml) into this channel in the hope that it will re-open. If this fails, then the following steps should be followed.

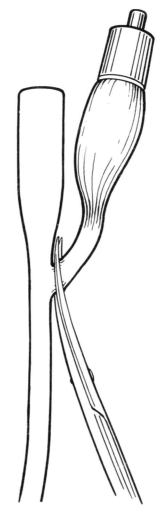

Fig. 10.6 Cut off the side arm of the catheter (not the central lumen).

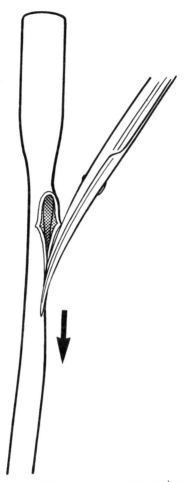

Fig. 10.7   If the water still does not appear, open up the second lumen
with scissors. Obtain additional length by gentle traction on the catheter.

If this fails, seek help. Do not believe that you can burst the balloon
either by over-distending it or by instilling noxious substances – neither
approach works and both are potentially dangerous. The safest method
of removal in men is direct puncture of the balloon with a spinal needle
through the abdominal wall under ultrasound control. In the female, the
balloon can be punctured through the anterior wall of the vagina, after
swabbing the vagina with chlorhexidene solution.

Suprapubic aspiration

Suprapubic aspiration of urine is occasionally necessary to diagnose urinary tract infection in both adults and children. The principles of the procedure are the same as for suprapubic catheterization, a syringe and needle replacing the catheter and trocar. A skin incision is unnecessary, but the skin should be infiltrated with local anaesthesia.

Suprapubic catheterization

This procedure should be performed only under the supervision of senior surgical staff under sterile conditions.

Position

The patient should be supine.

Equipment

(1) A suprapubic catheter (this usually comes in a set with an introducer)
(2) A scalpel (with a size 15 blade)
(3) A receiver
(4) A drainage bag.

Complications

Puncture of another intra-abdominal viscus (e.g. the small bowel) is very unlikely if the catheter is inserted when the bladder is full, because the full bladder displaces the peritoneum of the anterior abdominal wall upwards. This leaves no other intra-abdominal structure between the skin above the pubis and the lower part of the anterior surface of the bladder. Structures at the base of the bladder (such as the prostate) are in danger only if the catheter is inserted at an over-acute angle.

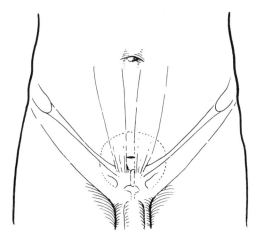

Fig. 10.8   After preparing and draping the suprapubic skin, inject local anaesthesia over a point 1–2 cm above the pubic bone in the midline. Make an incision (no more than 1 cm in length) through the skin and extend it down to the linea alba.

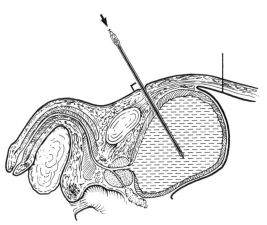

Fig. 10.9   Insert the suprapubic catheter with its trocar at right angles to the skin. A slight 'give' will be felt as it passes through the linea alba, and then again as it enters the bladder. A Malécot's catheter is demonstrated here with the tip stretched over the introducer to eliminate the bulb.

Fig. 10.10   Withdraw the trocar, allowing the tip to splay open and urine to be aspirated to confirm success. Insert the catheter as far as possible, so that when the bladder empties and contracts down into the pelvis, the catheter is not left behind in the prevesical space. Secure the catheter to the skin either with adhesive tape or, better, with a suture identical to the drain fixation stitch described under chest drainage (see p. 96).

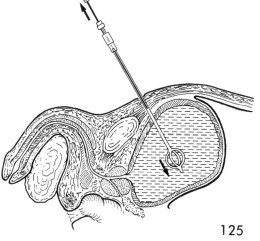

Vaginal examination

Examination of the female pelvis requires gentleness and tact. The patient must be relaxed and reassured to ensure maximum cooperation. Understanding the anatomical relations within the female pelvis and the ability to assess these is required in many specialties apart from gynaecology.

Position

The patient is supine with the ankles together, knees flexed and hips abducted, or in the left lateral position, as for rectal examination (see p. 114).

Equipment

(1) A glove and lubricant (jelly or obstetric cream)
(2) A speculum – a two-bladed, self-retracting (Cusco's) speculum is used when the patient is supine; when the patient is lying in the left lateral position, the single-bladed (Sims') speculum is more appropriate and allows assessment of both anterior and posterior vaginal wall prolapse in addition to uterine descent.

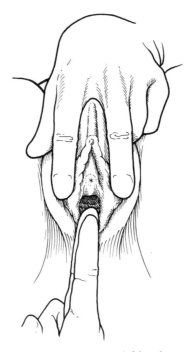

Fig. 10.11   If the patient is supine use the left hand to part the labia majora, and gently insert the index and middle finger of the right hand into the introitus, after first lubricating with jelly or obstetric cream. If the introitus is tight, as in a virgin, only the index figure should be inserted.

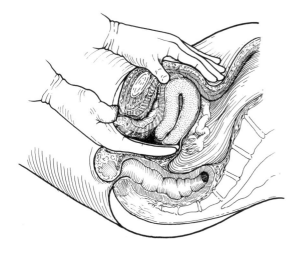

Fig. 10.12 Having identified the cervix with the fingers of the right hand, examine the adnexae by moving the fingers to each fornix while at the same time pressing downwards into each iliac fossa with the left hand. Both ovaries are normally easily palpable using this method, and any abnormalities of the tube are also detected.

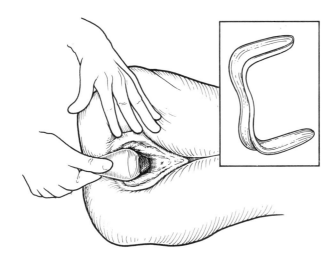

Fig. 10.13 Follow the same procedure if the patient is in the left lateral position, except use the left hand to raise the right buttock and labia majora before inserting the examining digits. Thereafter, palpate and compress the abdomen with the left hand as already described. This is a useful position from which to assess vaginal wall and uterine prolapse. Introduce a Sims' speculum (insert) into the vagina, and press it backwards to assess the anterior wall and forwards to assess the posterior wall.

TAKING A SMEAR

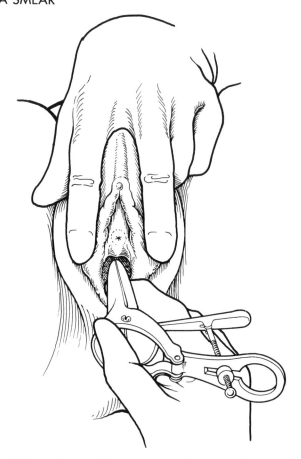

Fig. 10.14 After examining the cervix and fornices, withdraw the examining digits. Lubricate the blades of the Cusco's speculum and insert the speculum in the closed position with the handle facing sideways.

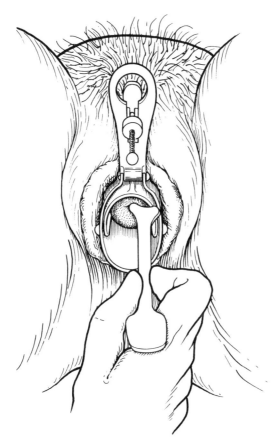

Fig. 10.15   When the blades have been inserted fully, turn the handle to point upwards. Now open the blades. Manipulation of the speculum will allow the cervix to be visualized between the blades. Insert the spatula into the vagina and the corner point into the cervical os. Rotate the spatula in a clockwise postion for 360°.

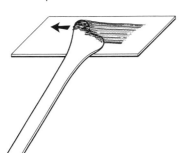

Fig. 10.16   After removal, wipe the spatula over the slide and place the slide immediately (to prevent air drying) into a smear pot containing a fixative of 95% alcohol solution (industrial methylated spirits BP). The slide must not be allowed to become air dried as this prevents subsequent cytological interpretation. It is recommended that you communicate with your local cytologist with regard to the preparation and fixation of the smear.

129

Nervous system

Lumbar puncture

Examination of a specimen of cerebrospinal fluid (CSF) is helpful in the diagnosis of a number of neurological conditions. The commonest indication is suspected meningitis. On no account should a lumbar puncture be performed in the presence of raised intracranial pressure (ICP). This procedure requires meticulous asepsis and the operator should be gowned, masked and gloved.

Position

If you are right-handed, put the patient on the left side with the knees drawn up to the chin. The shoulders and pelvis must be vertical to the floor; an assistant is helpful to maintain this position. Time spent achieving the correct position will make the rest of the procedure easier.

Equipment

(1) A spinal needle (18G)
(2) A CSF manometer with a three-way tap
(3) Specimen bottles for cell counts, glucose, protein and bacteriology.

Special points

(1) The needle must not be inserted more than 1 cm beyond the dura.
(2) Aspiration of CSF with a syringe should not be done.
(3) If the needle strikes bone on entry, withdraw it to the subcutaneous tissues and start again. If unsuccessful at the L3–L4 level, an attempt can be made at L2–L3 level.
(4) Queckenstedt's manoeuvre of compressing the internal jugular veins should show a rise in the ICP. Failure to demonstrate a rise indicates a spinal block above the needle. This manoeuvre is considered dangerous by some people and should not be performed routinely.

Complications

(1) Headache
(2) Dry tap
(3) Dural leak
(4) Meningitis
(5) Subdural, epidural or intrathecal haematoma
(6) Brain herniation (coning), when the brain becomes lodged in the foramen magnum and death occurs rapidly, as a result of rapid decompression from the lumbar puncture. This occurs when the ICP is high, and lumbar puncture should be avoided if there is a suspicion of raised ICP.

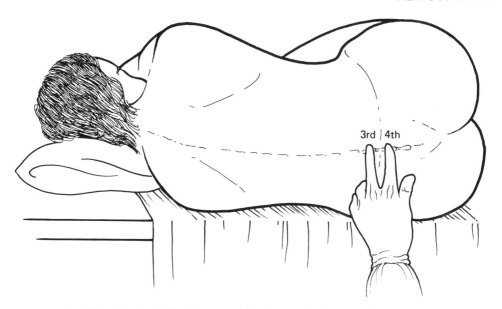

3rd | 4th

Fig. 11.1   Identify the L3–L4 interspace by drawing a line between the
highest points of the iliac crests. This line crosses the spinous processes of
L4. The aim is to go through the interspinous ligaments. Clean and drape
the skin. Infiltrate the skin and deep tissues with local anaesthetic at an
angle of 5–10° towards the head, as this is the direction of insertion.

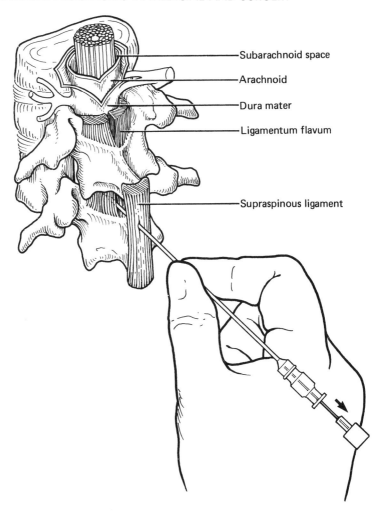

Fig. 11.2   Insert an 18G spinal needle through the skin at the angle described for Fig. 11.1, aiming to be parallel with the spinous processes. The needle should also be parallel to the floor. Because the needle is flexible and liable to bend, hold it between the forefinger and thumb a short distance from the skin. As the needle passes through the ligamentum flavum, you will feel a 'give'. Advance the needle slowly, and a further 'give' will be felt on going through the dura mater. Now advance the needle very slowly and withdraw the stylet every few millimetres. CSF will drip from the needle when the needle is in the correct place.

The feel of a 'give' going through the dura is difficult to sense, and it is advisable to withdraw the stylet every few millimetres after penetrating the ligamentum flavum.

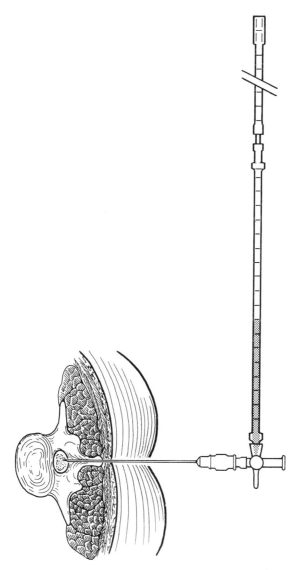

Fig. 11.3   When fluid is obtained, attach a manometer via a three-way tap for the measurement of pressure. Zero is the level of the needle. The fluid level in the manometer should rise and fall with respiration. Queckenstedt's manoeuvre (see above) can be done at this point. Collect three or four drops of CSF into each of three bottles for the measurement of cell count and differential, protein and glucose, and for bacteriology including serology. If blood is obtained, further serial samples must be taken. If the colour clears with time, then a traumatic puncture is likely.

:
:

Chapter 12

Aspiration/biopsy

Fine needle aspiration

Fine needle aspiration cytology can be used in the diagnosis of many diseases but is especially useful in attempts to distinguish benign from malignant disease. It is suitable for any lump or node in an accessible position, e.g. lymph nodes, thyroid, breast.

Position

The patient is placed in a comfortable supine position that allows you easy access to the lump.

Equipment

(1) A 20 ml syringe
(2) A 23G needle (21G for the breast)
(3) A slide or container (consult the local cytology department, particularly with respect to the use of millipore filters)
(4) A one-handed syringe handle (if available).

Special points

For making suitable slides, a single drop of aspirate is placed on the slide near the frosted end. The drop is then smeared across this slide with the smooth surface of another slide. It is usual to make approximately five slides. Some slides are fixed in alcohol and others are allowed to dry in air. This preparation is usually carried out by the cytologist. Alternatively, in some cytology departments, solid aspirates are ejected into 95% alcohol solution for transporting to the laboratory.

Complications

(1) An acellular specimen
(2) Haematoma formation
(3) Injury to local structures.

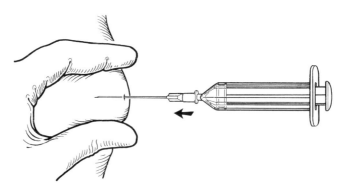

Fig. 12.1   After the skin is prepared, hold the lump to be needled immobile with the left hand, and with a rapid movement, insert the needle directly into the lump with the right hand.

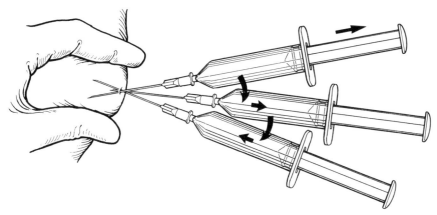

Fig. 12.2   Apply suction by pulling back on the syringe plunger. Keeping the suction on at all times, perform several back and forth movements in varying directions to ensure that a cellular aspirate is obtained. Should the lump be cystic, send the aspirated fluid in a specimen bottle directly to the laboratory. Gently release the vacuum with the needle still in the lump, so that pressure is equalized, and then remove the needle and syringe.

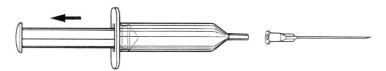

Fig. 12.3   Disconnect the needle from the syringe and fill the barrel with air.

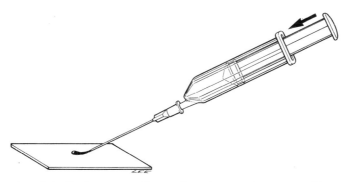

Fig. 12.4   Finally, reconnect the needle and express the contents of the needle either onto a slide or into a suitable fluid medium, as requested by the local cytology department.

Needle biopsy

The Tru-cut ® needle is the most widely used instrument for biopsy of tissue to obtain an adequate sample for histopathology. Any accessible tissue is suitable for such biopsy, although special precautions are necessary for certain organs, such as the liver, and advice should be taken from a senior colleague before attempting any biopsy. This section will describe the principles of using the needle for biopsy of a lump in the conventional manner, and the method used for biopsy of a breast lump. It is advisable to practise the manoeuvres with the needle before using it for the first time.

Position

The patient should be supine in a comfortable position that allows you easy access to the lump to be sampled.

Equipment

(1) A Tru-cut ® biopsy needle
(2) A specimen pot with fixative solution
(3) A scalpel with a size 11 blade
(4) A 21G needle.

Complications

(1) Haemorrhage or haematoma
(2) Local infection
(3) Injury to local structures
(4) Inconclusive histology.

THE TRU-CUT BIOPSY TECHNIQUE

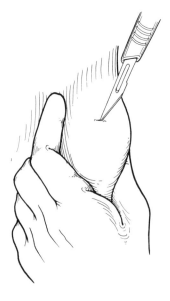

Fig. 12.5   Prepare the skin and infiltrate with local anaesthetic. Fix the lump with the fingers of the left hand. Make a small 2–3 mm incision through the skin with a scalpel because the needle is not designed for the penetration of skin.

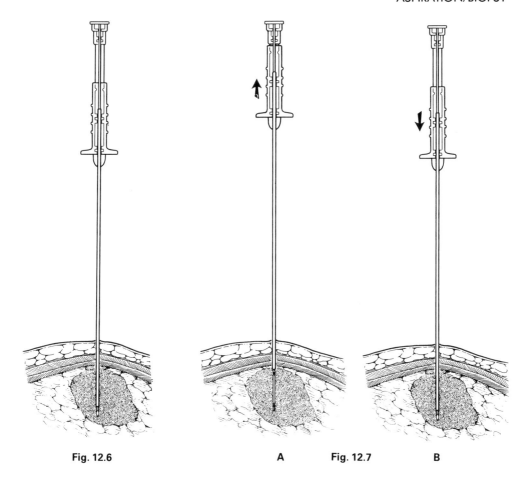

Fig. 12.6   A   **Fig. 12.7**   B

Fig. 12.6   Insert the needle into the lump with the specimen notch covered by the outer sleeve. You will need to operate the needle with two hands, and so once the lump has been penetrated by the needle, release the lump from your fingers or ask an assistant to hold it steady.

Fig. 12.7   Take the biopsy by withdrawing the outer sleeve, thus exposing the biopsy notch (A) and then advancing the outer sleeve over the trocar (B). Remove the entire needle in the closed position, as for insertion. Pick the specimen out of the gutter of the device with the 21G needle and transfer it to the fixative solution. Apply a small adhesive dressing.

TRU-CUT BIOPSY OF THE BREAST

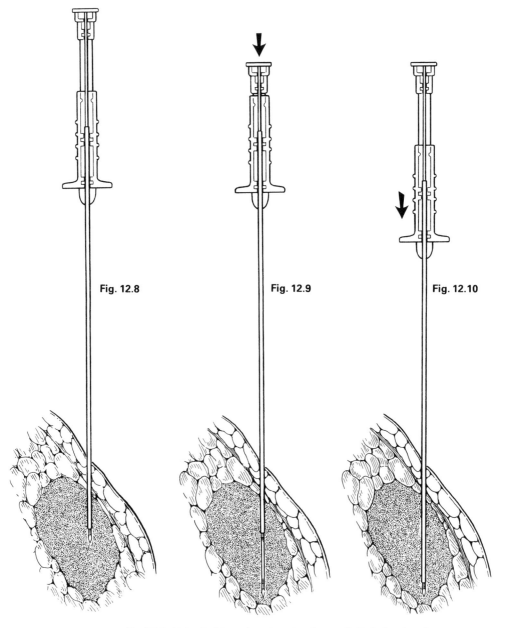

Fig. 12.8   Fig. 12.9   Fig. 12.10

Fig. 12.8   Take the biopsy by advancing the needle tip in the closed position into the lump.

Fig. 12.9   Advance the inner trocar into the lump.

Fig. 12.10   Advance the outer sleeve over the inner trocar and withdraw the needle in the closed position.

TRU CUT BIOPSY OF THE LIVER

This procedure should be carried out only after adequate personal instruction and with supervision. There are several pre-biopsy investigations that must be done to ensure safety: a full blood count, clotting screen and blood group with serum save.

Position

The patient should be lying supine with the right side adjacent to the edge of the bed. The right arm is rested above the head.

Equipment

(1) A Tru-cut ® needle
(2) A specimen pot with fixative. Occasionally a special medium will be required for a particular investigation.

Management

The patient is left lying on the right side for two to three hours, and then in a supine position for four hours. During this time, regular (half-hourly) observations of pulse and blood pressure should be done. Bed rest should continue for 24 hours and regular (two-hourly) observations taken. The aim of such rigorous observation is to identify early signs of haemorrhage that will require resuscitation and possibly surgery to control.

Complications

(1) Haemorrhage
(2) Cholangitis
(3) Biliary peritonitis
(4) Puncture of the kidney, colon and gall bladder
(5) Pneumothorax/haemothorax.

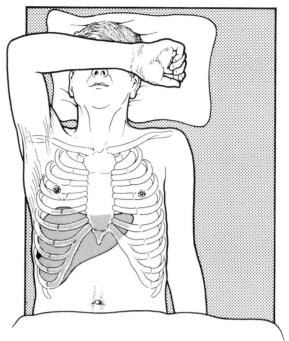

Fig. 12.11 The site of insertion lies between the anterior and mid-axillary lines of the intercostal space one below where there is maximum dullness to percussion on full expiration. This is usually the eighth, ninth or tenth space.

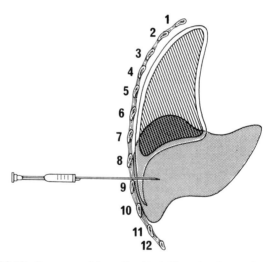

Fig. 12.12 Prepare and drape the skin. Infiltrate local anaesthetic down to and including the liver capsule. Incise the skin with a scalpel. Pass the needle over the top of the rib to avoid injury to the intercostal neurovascular bundle, and insert it up to the liver edge. Tell the patient to take a deep breath, exhale and hold the breath (it is wise to practise this beforehand with the patient). Advance the needle into the right lobe of the liver for about 4–5 cm and take the biopsy as described for Figs. 12.6 and 12.7. The moment the needle is withdrawn, the patient can start breathing again.

Chapter 13

Minor operations

Minor operations on the skin, appendages and subcutaneous tissue

The procedures that will be discussed here may be carried out on the ward or within the confines of the A & E or outpatient department under local anaesthesia. They are performed under aseptic conditions, and the surgeon should be gloved but not necessarily gowned. The only possible exception to this is lymph node biopsy, which is best carried out in the operating theatre under general anaesthetic.

Position

The area involving the lesion is well exposed. If the arm is involved, this should be positioned on an appropriate rest with the hand in the functional position.

Equipment

(1) A scalpel and a fine blade (usually size 15)
(2) Fine toothed forceps
(3) Dissecting scissors
(4) A needle holder
(5) Suture scissors
(6) A McDonald's elevator for procedures on the toe-nails
(7) A self-retaining retractor for lymph node biopsy.

EXCISION OF A SKIN LESION

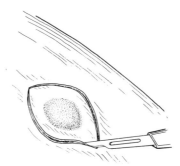

Fig. 13.1 Infiltrate local anaesthesia around the lesion, as demonstrated earlier (see p. 24), and make an elliptical incision, preferably so that the long axis lies parallel to the skin creases of that region. The 'clearance' around the lesion, both radially and in depth, will depend on its nature, potentially malignant lesions requiring a wider margin (5–10 mm) than benign naevi.

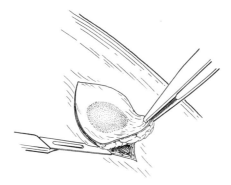

Fig. 13.2 Use toothed forceps to grasp one end of the ellipse, and then mobilize the ellipse from the subcutaneous tissue. The deep plane of dissection is through the layer of subcutaneous fat.

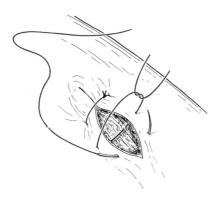

Fig. 13.3 Close the elliptical defect using interrupted nylon sutures.

EXCISION OF A SEBACEOUS CYST

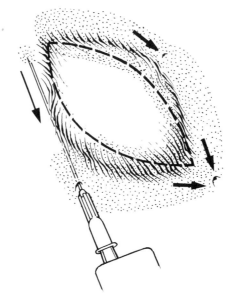

Fig. 13.4 After preparing the skin, infiltrate local anaesthesia around the cyst. If injected into the correct plane (between the cyst wall and the subcutaneous tissue), it will assist in isolating the cyst from the surrounding tissue, making subsequent dissection easier.

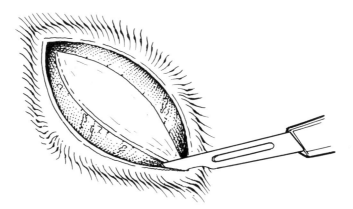

Fig. 13.5 Make a narrow elliptical incision over the cyst along the lines of the surrounding skin creases. This 'island' of skin will be useful for grasping later in the procedure, thus minimizing the possibility of puncturing the cyst which carries the risk of leaving a small portion behind to produce a recurrence.

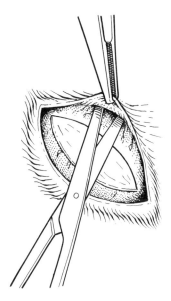

Fig. 13.6   Grasp the edges of the wound with fine toothed forceps and mobilize the cyst by blunt dissection using curved dissecting scissors (artery forceps are a substitute) inserted into the plane between the cyst and the surrounding skin.

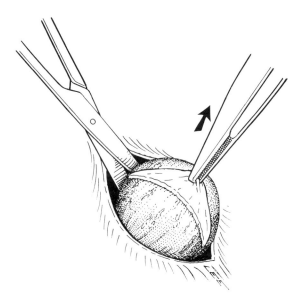

Fig. 13.7   Once the cyst has been mobilized on all sides, grasp the central skin ellipse and free the undersurface of the cyst, preferably with sharp dissection. Failure to remove all of the cyst wall is likely to result in recurrence, and so if the cyst is burst, make an extra effort to remove the remaining cyst wall. Close the wound with interrupted nylon sutures.

149

EXCISION OF A LYMPH NODE

This is best performed in the operating theatre under general anaesthesia. Lymph nodes removed for diagnostic decisions should be divided into two pieces; one is placed in formal saline for histological examination, and the second is placed in sterile normal saline and sent for bacteriological investigation – which will usually include culture for tuberculosis.

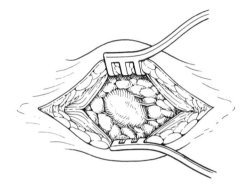

Fig. 13.8   Make at least a 2 cm incision over the lymph node along Langer's lines, and extend it down into the subcutaneous fat. Insert a self-retaining retractor and expose the lymph node by blunt dissection.

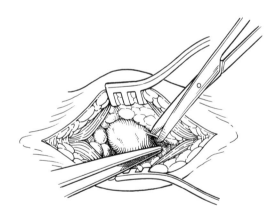

Fig. 13.9   Once the lymph node has been found, mobilize it from the surrounding tissue without grasping it. This prevents distortion which makes subsequent histological examination difficult. Use dissecting forceps to push the surrounding tissue away from the lymph node, and free the node by sharp dissection. Ligate large afferent or efferent vessels. Insert two or three absorbable subcutaneous sutures if the dead space is large, and close the wound with a single layer of interrupted nylon sutures.

REMOVAL OF A TOE-NAIL

Management

The dressing should be left in situ until it drops off. Repeated changing is not only painful for the patient but will disrupt all the newly formed granulation tissue. If it remains past seven days, it will usually detach itself after soaking in warm water.

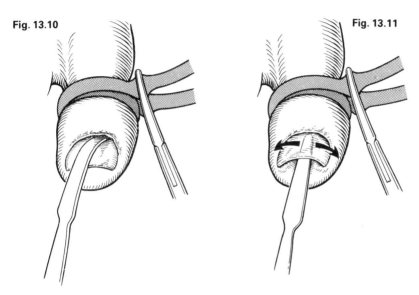

Fig. 13.10 **Fig. 13.11**

Fig. 13.10   After cleaning the foot and digits thoroughly, drape the foot to expose the great toe and perform a digital block (see p. 30). Once adequate anaesthesia has been achieved, and this may take at least five minutes, apply a tourniquet to the base of the toe, as illustrated. Pull a thin rubber tube tightly around the base of the digit and clamp the two ends with artery forceps. Push the cuticle of the nail proximally and, if possible, free it from the upper surface of the nail using the curved end of a McDonald's elevator. This will facilitate the later removal of the nail.

Fig. 13.11   Insert the flat end of the McDonald's elevator under the nail and advance it proximally while at the same time sweeping it from side to side, lifting the nail from the nail bed and separating it from the skin at each side. Continue this procedure until the whole nail lies free. It is important to extend the blunt dissection up to the distal interphalangeal joint proximally, to ensure that the nail is completely freed from the nail bed.

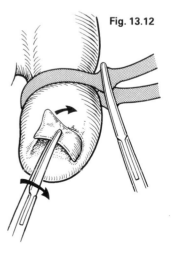

Fig. 13.12

Fig. 13.12   Grasp the nail with artery forceps and remove it by twisting to one side, as shown. At this stage, the cuticle may still require to be detached from the upper surface of the nail by sharp dissection. Clean the wound with antiseptic solution and dress it with paraffin gauze followed by dry gauze. Finally, release the tourniquet.

WEDGE RESECTION OF A TOE-NAIL

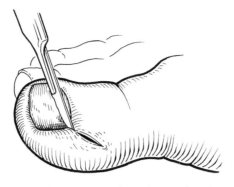

Fig. 13.13 Prepare the great toe as for nail removal. Make an incision (approximately 1 cm) in the angle of the nail on the side to be removed (medial in this diagram) using a size 15 blade, and extend it down to the nail.

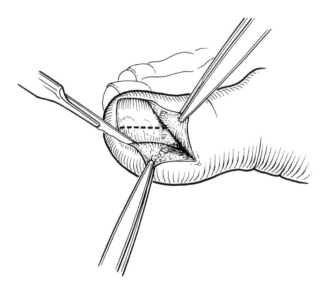

Fig. 13.14 Raise the skin from the nail on both sides of the incision by sharp dissection, and cut the nail longitudinally as indicated by the dotted line.

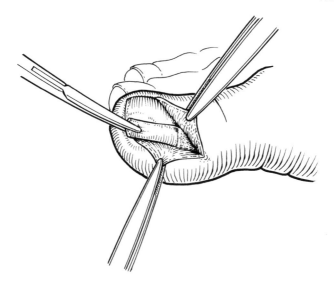

Fig. 13.15   Separate the required portion of the nail from the nail bed using the McDonald's elevator, and remove it with artery forceps.

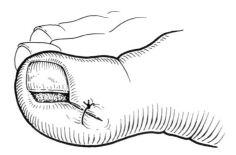

Fig. 13.16   Suture the wound at the angle of the nail bed with a single 3/0 nylon suture, and then dress it.

NAIL BED EXCISION

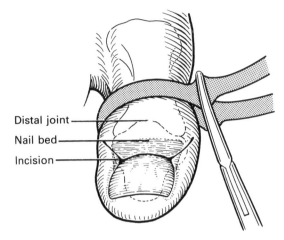

Distal joint —
Nail bed —
Incision —

Fig. 13.17 The nail bed lies beneath the proximal part of the nail and extends proximally to the distal interphalangeal joint. It is shown here by the shaded area. Prepare the great toe as described previously, and make two incisions at the angles of the nail, extending them down to the nail.

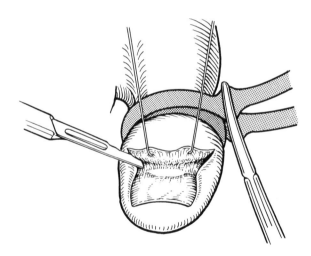

Fig. 13.18 Raise the skin proximal to the nail by sharp dissection until the proximal extent of the nail bed is seen. Lift the nail and remove it as described previously.

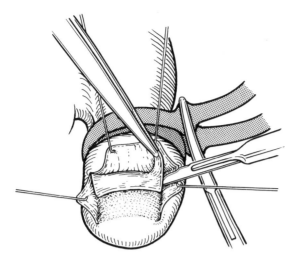

Fig. 13.19   Now mobilize the germinal part of the nail bed. First, free it from the distal phalanx by a transverse incision made just distal to the distal interphalangeal joint down to the underlying bone. Extend this at each corner around the side of the phalanx and then complete it by a distal transverse incision at the level of the cuticle. Take care not to enter the joint capsule and also to ensure that all germinal tissue at the corners of the incision are removed. This will prevent the problem of recurrent nail spicules.

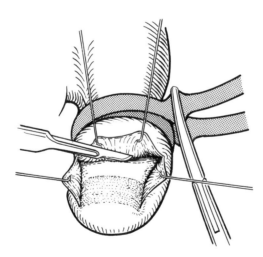

Fig. 13.20   Remove the whole germinal part of the nail bed from the underlying bone by sharp dissection. Suture the corners of the wound with a single 3/0 nylon suture, and dress the wound as before.

DRAINAGE OF AN ABSCESS

The only correct management for an abscess is drainage. Antibiotic therapy has no place in the treatment of a fully established abscess unless there is concomitant cellulitis or lymphangitis. Drainage of abscesses is best performed under general anaesthesia in the operating room, although small subcutaneous ones may be drained in the A & E or outpatient department after anaesthetizing the surrounding skin with ethyl chloride spray. Lignocaine should not be injected into infected tissues; increased absorption into the systemic circulation may occur leading to possible dangerous side-effects (see p. 23). Peri-operative antibiotics are only required in special circumstances – such as occur with previous rheumatic heart disease, the presence of prostheses (e.g. a hip replacement, central lines etc.) or signs of immune deficiency – when bacterial 'seeding' is particularly hazardous. In such circumstances, antibiotics active against the suspected organism should be given with the premedication.

Position

The patient is placed in such a position as to allow maximum exposure of the infected area.

Equipment

(1)   A scalpel and a size 10 blade
(2)   Toothed forceps
(3)   Curved Mayo scissors
(4)   Sinus forceps
(5)   1" ribbon gauze
(6)   Proflavin solution.

Management

Dressings should be changed daily, with care being taken to fill the wound down to its deepest aspect. This will allow it to heal from the bottom upwards, preventing recurrence.

Complications

Damage to surrounding structures following injudicious use of the knife. This is more common in regions such as the perineum where abscesses are often closely associated with important surrounding structures.

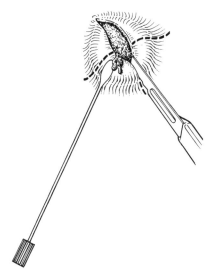

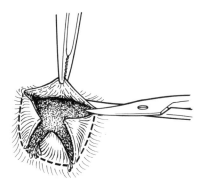

Fig. 13.22 Pick up the edges of the cruciate incision with toothed forceps and excise them using the Mayo scissors. This converts the incision from a star into a hole and will prevent premature closing of the wound in the early postoperative period.

Fig. 13.21 After preparing and draping the area of the abscess, make a cruciate incision, as shown. A bacteriological swab must be taken from the pus immediately after incision.

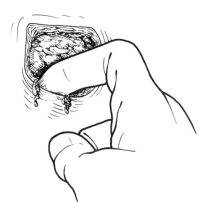

Fig. 13.23 Break down loculations within the abscess cavity with the index finger, ensuring that no part remains undrained.

Fig. 13.24 Soak 1″ ribbon gauze in proflavin and insert it into the wound, starting in the deepest part and working superficially. Place a light dressing over the wound and secure it with elastoplast.

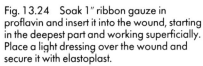

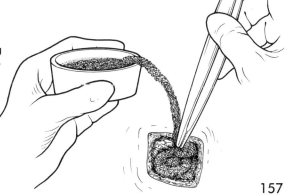

Orthopaedics

Plaster casts

Plaster of Paris remains the standard method for external splintage of an injured limb. Its application is truly a case of 'it looks easier than it is'. Great care must be taken to avoid any of the disastrous complications that can follow application of plaster casts.

Position

The limb to be plastered should be completely supported in the position desired. This usually means having an assistant.

Equipment

(1) Plaster of Paris bandages (these come in several widths – common sense dictates which size to use)
(2) A bucket of tepid water
(3) Waterproof sheets and aprons
(4) Plaster shears
(5) Stockinette
(6) Orthopaedic wool bandages

Special points

(1) The warmer the water, the quicker the plaster will harden – and also the higher the temperature generated during this process.
(2) There are no definite indicators that a plaster has hardened and it is a good idea to count to 10 after you think the plaster has set before letting go.

Management

(1) Plaster takes 48 hours to dry out and set completely, and so it must be protected until this time: slings for the upper limb and crutches for the lower limb.
(2) Plaster needs to be protected from water.
(3) Pain, changes in sensation, cold digits, loss of movement, cyanosis or pallor must be reported early by the patient and, if there is any suggestion of a circulatory obstruction, the plaster must be split or 'bivalved' (cut into two halves). Splitting means every layer down to the skin, not just the plaster. For this reason, it is often better to use plaster slabs or split casts in a fresh injury where swelling is likely.

Complications

(1) Local skin necrosis
(2) Pressure neuropathies
(3) Circulatory obstruction leading to amputation or ischaemic contracture
(4) Joint deformity
(5) Joint stiffness.

USING PLASTER OF PARIS BANDAGES

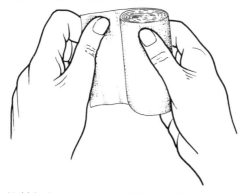

Fig. 14.1   Hold the bandage in the right hand with a few centimetres unrolled and the end in the left hand. Submerge the bandage in the bucket with both hands. Allow the air bubbles to escape, and give a gentle squeeze to the roll to express the last bubbles. Do not squeeze tightly, as this will cause difficulty in manipulating the plaster.

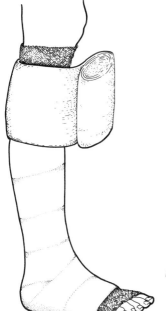

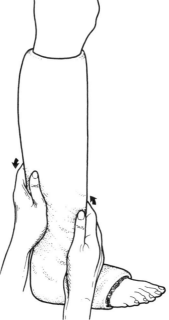

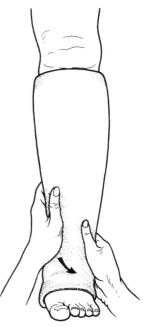

Fig. 14.2   Now roll the bandage onto the limb using both hands; do not pull it on like a conventional crêpe bandage. Each revolution should overlap the previous one by a third, and each bandage should be rolled in one direction only. If specific reinforcement is necessary, it is best to use a plaster slab which is held in position by the plaster bandage being rolled around it.

Fig. 14.3   To smooth the plaster, use the palm of the hands and rub them over the plaster in the same direction as the plaster was rolled on – any other way will just create dangerous ridges in the plaster. Do this with every roll applied, as it helps bonding between layers.

Fig. 14.4   To mould the plaster, wait until it is beginning to harden and then apply pressure over the required point(s) with the palm of the hand; this pressure must be kept up until the plaster has set. Avoid fingers which dig into the plaster. Correct moulding is the secret to providing a cast that will 'do the job'. Beauty comes with experience!

161

APPLICATION OF A PLASTER CAST

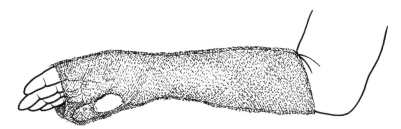

Fig. 14.5   Cut the stockinette to the correct length, which is 5 cm longer than the cast at either end, and roll it onto the limb. Cut holes for thumbs as necessary.

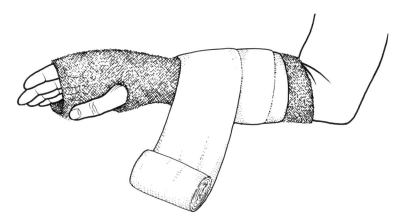

Fig. 14.6   Roll on the wool bandage starting from one end and making sure that no ridges appear. Overlap the bandage by one third. Extra padding is necessary at prominent bony points and at sites where pressure will be applied for moulding.

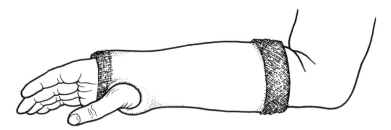

Fig. 14.7   Apply the plaster as described above. Before putting on the last roll, turn back the stockinette and smooth it onto the wet plaster. Carefully cover the stockinette with the last roll. Do any necessary moulding and hold it until the plaster has hardened.

REMOVING A PLASTER CAST

With shears

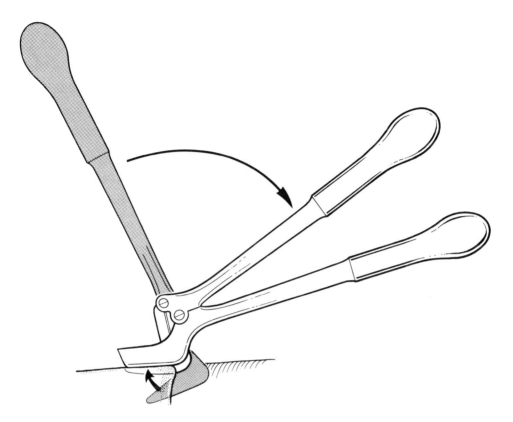

Fig. 14.8   Plan the line of your cut, avoiding bony points and wounds. It is sensible in certain areas to bivalve the plaster to remove it, rather than making a single cut. The shears must be used correctly to avoid injury to the skin. Hold the lower handle steady with the blade parallel to the plaster; use the upper handle for the cutting motion. Advance the shears gently for a few centimetres after each cut. The shears frequently become clogged with debris, particularly if a large amount of padding has been used; when this happens, remove the shears and clean the blades. It is better to use a pair of blunt-nosed scissors to cut the underlying padding and stockinette. As you proceed along the plaster, widen the cut with the plaster separators or with your hands, so that you can get to the soft padding. When the entire plaster has been cut down to the skin, gently part the two edges until the limb can be lifted out. Remember that the limb will be atrophied and the joints stiff making full control difficult, so help the patient by holding the limb initially.

With a plaster saw

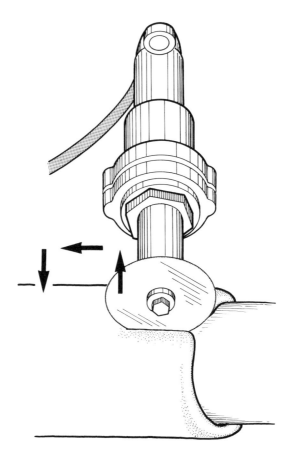

Fig. 14.9   The saw acts by an oscillating movement and will not cut the skin if applied directly to it; however, it is easy to injure the skin if the saw is dragged along it, and so correct technique is important. Push the saw directly down onto the plaster – a 'give' will be felt as you go through to the padding. Then lift the saw up, move it along and use the same downward pressure. On no account should the saw be used in a horizontal cutting action.

Insertion of skeletal traction pins

This procedure can be performed under local or general anaesthetic. Sterile conditions and technique are desirable, although it is not essential for the procedure to be carried out in an operating theatre; it may be necessary to do this in the A & E department.

Position

The patient is positioned supine with the leg supported by sandbags.

Equipment

(see Figs. 14.10 and 14.11)
(1) Traction pins, which come in several lengths and widths and are of two general types: unthreaded (e.g. Steinmann) and threaded (e.g. Denham)
(2) A hand drill with a chuck key
(3) Pin hooks and guards
(4) A stirrup
(5) A scalpel with a size 15 blade
(6) An image intensifier if any manipulation is to be performed.

Complications

(1) Skin necrosis
(2) Malposition of a pin
(3) Pin track infection
(4) Pin loosening
(5) Injury to the opposite leg.

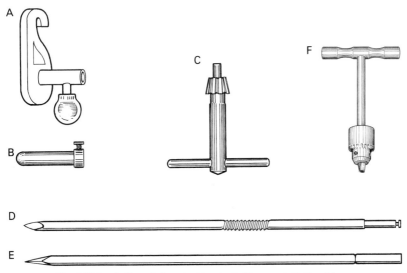

Fig. 14.10   A. Simonis R; swivel hooks; B. Pin guard; C. Chuck key;
D. Denham pin; E. Steinmann pin; F. Hand bit.

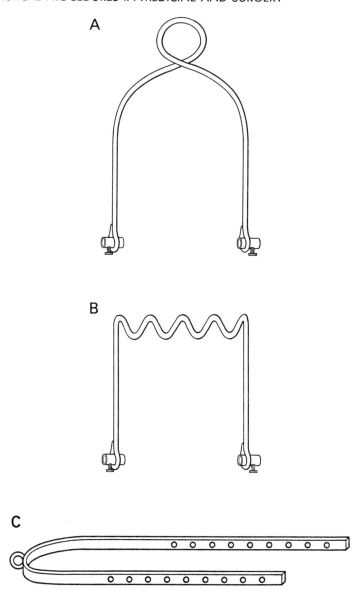

Fig. 14.11   Three types of stirrup which can be attached to the pin following insertion.

INSERTION OF AN UPPER TIBIAL PIN

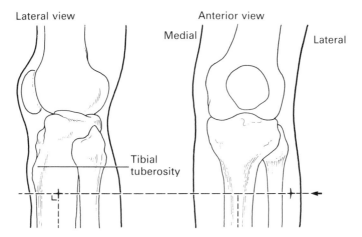

Fig. 14.12   The correct site for insertion of an upper tibial pin is just distal to the tibial tubercle, 2.5 cm below the anterior border of the tibia. Mark the sites of entry and exit with an indelible marker, and prepare and drape the skin. Infiltrate local anaesthetic down to and including the periosteum at both the entry and exit sites. Always insert the pin from lateral to medial, and make a small cruciate incision at the point of entry. Advance the pin loaded in the chuck to the lateral cortex. With a twisting to-and-fro motion, breach the cortex and advance the pin towards the medial cortex.

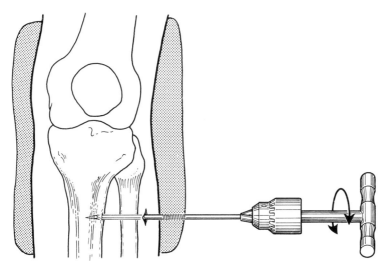

Fig. 14.13   It is very important to ensure that the pin is aligned accurately at 90° to the long axis of the leg and parallel to the floor while advancing it through the bone.

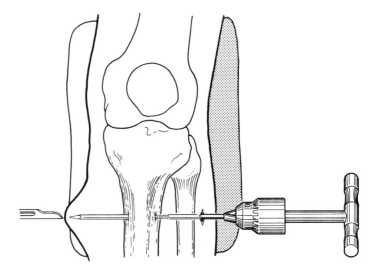

Fig. 14.14   A firm grip on the leg with the opposite hand is essential for accurate placement. Continue the twisting motion until the medial cortex is breached; advance the pin further until the skin is tented. Make a cruciate incision over this point, and advance the pin so that equal lengths protrude. If a threaded pin is used, engage the thread in the lateral cortex by turning the pin in a clockwise direction.

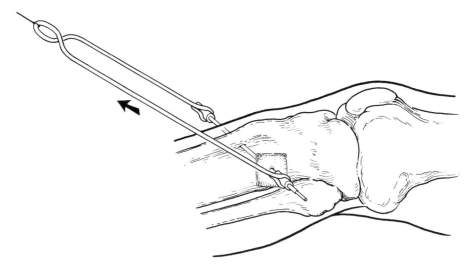

Fig. 14.15   Dress the wounds and apply a crêpe bandage. Attach the stirrup or hooks and cover the ends of the pin with the guards.

INSERTION OF CALCANEAN PIN

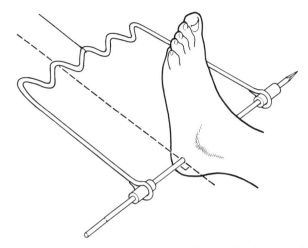

Fig. 14.16   Use the same preparation, anaesthesia and technique as for a tibial pin. The site of insertion is at a point midway down a vertical line from the tip of the lateral malleolus to the border of the heel. Insert the pin from lateral to medial, at 90° to the long axis of the leg and parallel to the floor to avoid the posterior tibial vessels. Use an unthreaded pin because the cortex of the calcaneus is thin and will not hold a thread. A K-wire is sufficient in most cases.

Setting up traction

Setting up traction requires an ability to tie knots and to follow simple diagrams. It is usual to set up the traction on the ward where all the necessary equipment should be available and the knowledge of the trained nursing staff can be sought; however, it is preferable to set traction up in the theatre recovery room if this is possible. Selection of weights and the positioning of the leg on traction need to be decided on an individual basis.

Equipment

(1) Traction cord
(2) Weights
(3) Pulleys
(4) Bed attachments.

Complications

The complications encountered are the same as for knee joint aspiration.

Management

Daily care involves: (1) Checking the pin sites
(2) Adjusting padding, pulleys and weights to keep correct alignment
(3) Checking for pressure areas.

Complications

(1) Malposition of a fracture leading to malunion
(2) Over-distraction leading to delayed union or non-union
(3) Pressure necrosis
(4) Nerve injury from both over-distraction and pressure
(5) Joint stiffness.

TRACTION FOR FEMORAL FRACTURES

Preparation of a Thomas splint

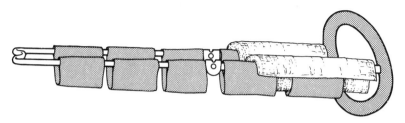

Fig. 14.17   Select a splint to fit the patient by measuring the length of the leg and circumference of the thigh of the uninjured side remembering to allow for swelling when considering circumference. Slings made from domette bandage are covered with gamgee and attached to the splint, as shown. If a Pearson knee piece is used (see Fig. 14.19 below), remember to prepare this in the same way and leave the rest of the Thomas splint free distal to its attachment.

Types of traction

There are many varieties of traction described for the management of femoral fractures with a tibial pin *in situ*. The following figures demonstrate four of the more common types.

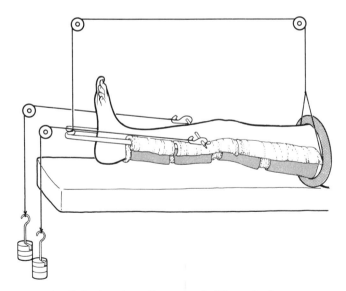

Fig. 14.18   Skeletal traction with a suspended Thomas' splint.

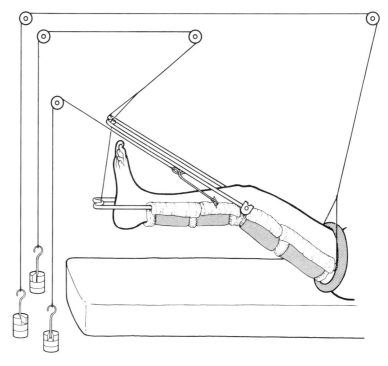

Fig. 14.19   Sliding skeletal traction with a Pearson knee piece.

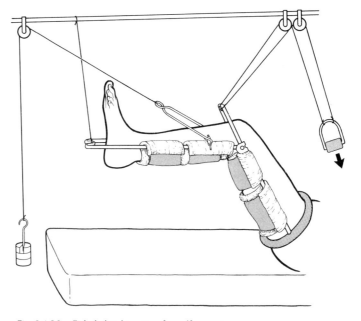

Fig. 14.20   Fisk skeletal traction for self-exercise.

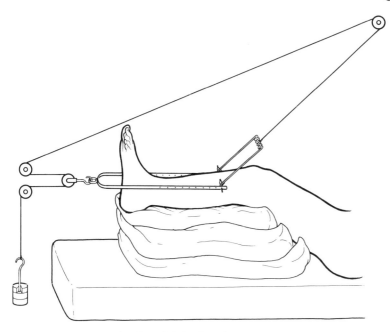

Fig. 14.21   Hamilton Russell skeletal traction.

TRACTION OF THE LOWER LEG

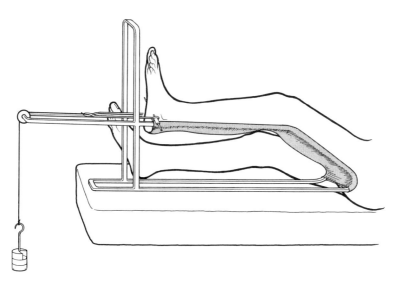

Fig. 14.22   For fractures of the lower leg on traction with a calcanean pin, rest the leg either on pillows or on a Bohler-Braun frame, as the diagram illustrates.

173

Joint aspiration

Aspiration of a joint is used for both diagnostic and therapeutic purposes. It is preferable to perform joint aspiration under sterile conditions to avoid any possibility of introducing infection. The knee and elbow joints are described, but the principles apply to any joint.

KNEE JOINT ASPIRATION

Position

The patient should be lying on his or her back with the leg extended and supported by sandbags as necessary.

Equipment
(1) An 18G needle
(2) A three-way tap
(3) A 20 ml syringe
(4) Specimen tubes.

Complications
(1) Infection
(2) Injury to intra-articular structures.

ELBOW JOINT ASPIRATION

This procedure is performed to relieve the pain caused by distension of the joint by blood following an intra-articular fracture, most commonly a fracture of the radial head.

Position

The patient should be sitting with the elbow at 90° and the forearm pronated. The arm should be resting comfortably on a table.

Equipment
(1) A 21G needle
(2) A three-way tap
(3) A 10 ml syringe.

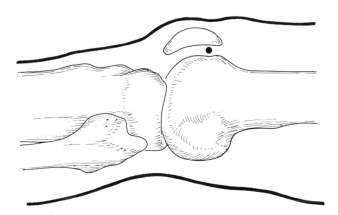

Fig. 14.23 Insert the needle on the lateral aspect of the knee beneath the upper pole of the patella. This point is 1 cm lateral to the edge of the patella and approximately 1 cm below its lower border.

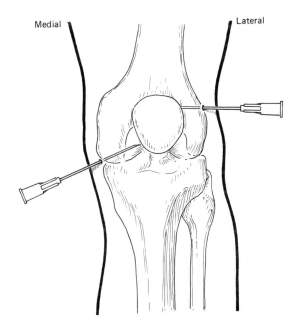

Medial

Lateral

Fig. 14.24 Ensure that the needle is inserted parallel to the floor in order to avoid injuring the articular cartilage. Should resistance be felt, withdraw the needle slightly and attempt a different angle. Avoid prodding the needle around the joint to obtain the last few millilitres of fluid. Attaching a three-way tap to the needle allows the syringe to be disconnected and emptied more easily. Send any fluid collected to the laboratory for microbiology and crystallography. An alternative approach to the joint is from the medial side. Insert the needle at the level of the joint line 1 cm medial to the edge of the patella. Keep the needle parallel to the floor and aim it a few degrees headward into the intercondylar notch. Again, try to avoid injuring the articular cartilage.

175

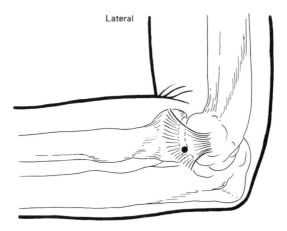

Fig. 14.25   Insert the needle between the lateral epicondyle and radial head. To find the joint line, gently rotate the forearm while palpating over the lateral aspect of the elbow; this will identify the radial head which can be felt rotating beneath your fingers and the joint line lies immediately proximally. (Identify these landmarks on yourself.)

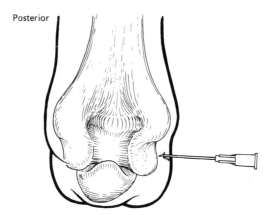

Fig. 14.26   Ensure that the needle is inserted medially and parallel to the floor. Aspirate with advancement. It is usual to obtain 5–20 ml of fluid.

Index